Portal Design
in Radiation
Therapy

Portal Design in Radiation Therapy

Byron G. Dasher, M.D.
Nancy H. Wiggers, M.D.
Anne Marie Vann, M.Ed., R.T.(R)(T)

Illustrations by Kirah L. Van Sickle, M.S.M.I.

 The R.L. Bryan Company

Byron G. Dasher, MD
Radiation Oncology Associates
Georgia Radiation Therapy Center
Augusta, Georgia

Nancy H. Wiggers, MD
Department of Radiation Oncology
Saint Joseph's Hospital
Atlanta, Georgia

Anne Marie Vann, M.Ed, RT(R)(T)
Program Director, Radiation Therapy Technology
Medical College of Georgia
Augusta, Georgia

© 1994 DWV Enterprises

Printed in the United States of America

ISBN 0-9642715-0-8

Library of Congress Catalog Card Number: 94-72510

The R. L. Bryan Company
301 Greystone Executive Park
P.O. Drawer 368
Columbia, S.C. 29202

Preface

It was the intent of the authors to design a textbook that can be used by radiation therapists and oncologists as a quick reference when simulating treatment portals. With the realization that a portal must be designed for each individual patient, the authors have described typical treatment portals to provide a guideline for simulation and treatment. For the unusual circumstances, the anatomy and primary routes of spread are discussed to allow the reader to tailor treatment portals based on the anatomical facts. This text includes only those sites where radiation is traditionally indicated in the patient's management.

Table of Contents

Chapter 1

Head and Neck Cancer

TREATMENT OF THE NECK

Treatment of the lymph nodes in primary head and neck cancers depends on many factors:
1) the site of primary disease (nasopharyngeal and pyriform sinus have a rich capillary lymphatic network as opposed to paranasal sinus, middle ear and vocal cords that have no capillary lymphatics)
2) the extent of primary disease (lymph node metastases increase with depth of invasion and extension into sites with rich capillary lymphatics)
3) size of the primary tumor (except for tumors of the nasopharynx and pyriform sinus which metastasize independent of tumor size)
4) cell type and differentiation (the more poorly differentiated, the greater the risk of lymph node metastases)
5) lymphatic vascular space invasion of the tumor
6) the clinical, or present nodal status of the patient

Anatomy

The first echelon of lymph nodes are usually included in the treatment portal encompassing the primary tumor. The lower neck is generally treated through a separate anterior neck portal when there is macroscopic or a risk for microscopic disease in this area. The lymph node regions that will be discussed in this chapter are diagrammed in Fig. 1.1.

Note that there are no posterior cervical nodes located behind the spinous processes.

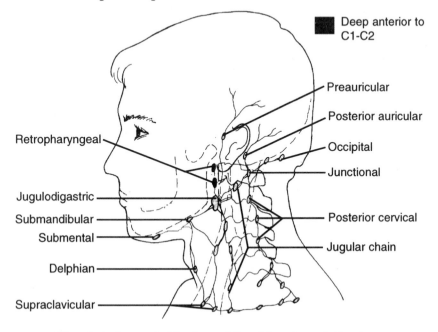

Fig. 1.1 Lymph Nodes of the Head and Neck

Treatment

Two parallel opposed lateral neck portals are utilized for midline tumors with a high incidence of nodal spread (nasopharynx, oropharynx, hypopharynx, supraglottic larynx). Well lateralized lesions may require only ipsilateral neck treatment (tonsillar region, retromolar trigone). Patients with prior neck surgery may have rerouting of lymphatics; and therefore, must have bilateral neck treatment.

Technical Aspects of Radiation Therapy

To treat a three field head and neck (an anterior, and two lateral ports), the patient is positioned supine. A head cushion that aligns the cervical spine should be used. (If the curve in the cervical spine is diminished, it is easier to reduce the port off of the spinal cord when high doses must be delivered). The patient's shoulders must be down and out of the lateral treatment field. If the lower cervical nodes must be included in the lateral treatment portals, it may be necessary to angle the treatment couch to encompass the nodes without treating the shoulders.

For tumors of the oral cavity, oropharynx, and nasopharynx, the junction of the lateral fields and the anterior neck portal should be at the thyroid notch. A block is placed in the anterior port to shield the larynx and spinal cord. The tracheal stoma should be electively treated in the anterior field in patients who have had an emergency tracheostomy, who exhibit subglottic extension, close or positive margins, or involvement of the soft tissues of the neck.

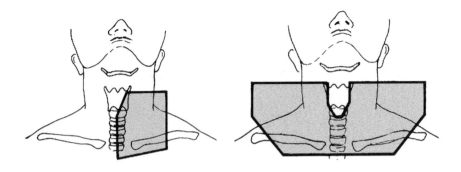

Fig. 1.2a Lower Neck Field for
        Well Lateralized Lesions

Fig. 1.2b Anterior Neck Field

If the primary lesion extends below the thyroid notch, the junction of the anterior and lateral port must be inferior to the primary lesion. In this case, you can no longer block the larynx in the anterior field. A small spinal cord block may be placed in the lateral fields, or in the anterior portal.

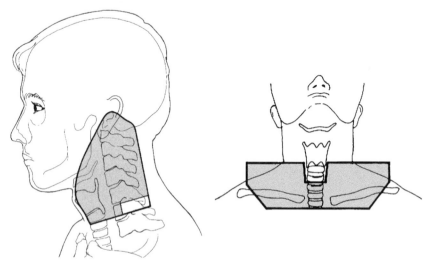

Fig. 1.3a Lateral Neck Port   Fig. 1.3b Anterior Neck Port

Most centers use a half-beam block at the junction of the anterior and lateral ports to prevent overlap of the fields. If the central ray is not utilized at the match line, then the collimator must be angled on the lateral fields to match the beam divergence from the anterior field. Spinal cord blocks should always be added in either the anterior or lateral fields to assure that the beams did not overlap in this area. The lateral fields are usually reduced off of the spinal cord at 45 Gy. When the posterior cervical nodes are at risk, they may be boosted with electrons to increase the dose to the nodes while sparing the spinal cord from additional radiation.

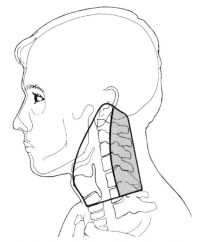

Fig. 1.4 Posterior Electron Port

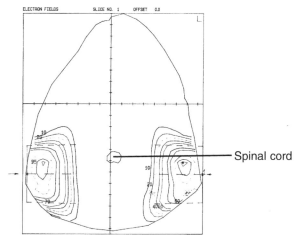

Fig. 1.5   9 MeV Electron Dose Distribution

Dose

A clinically negative neck (no evidence of nodal disease), which is at risk for subclinical disease, is effectively managed with radiation alone. Doses of 50 Gy at 1.8-2.0 Gy per fraction are recommended. This is advantageous compared to a radical neck dissection because it offers coverage of all nodal areas treated and there is less disfigurement.

In neck nodes that are treated postoperatively, slightly higher doses may be needed, due to changes in the blood supply (less oxygen carrying blood for free radical formation). Clinically positive nodes measuring ≤2 cm should be treated to 60 Gy, 2-3 cm nodes should be boosted to 70 Gy. In general, for nodes greater than 3 cm, preoperative or postoperative radiation is used.

Patients with borderline unresectable nodes should have the lymph nodes boosted to 60-80 Gy, and resection should follow after radiation therapy.

ORAL CAVITY

Oral cavity tumors account for less than 5% of all carcinomas in the United States. Over 80% of oral cavity tumors are keratinizing squamous cell carcinomas. Non-keratinizing squamous cell and minor salivary gland tumors are also found in this area. Basal cell carcinomas may arise from the skin of the lip.

Carcinoma of the lip constitutes about 45%, the oral tongue 17%, and the floor of the mouth 12%, of all oral cavity malignancies. Patients that smoke, consume alcohol, or who have poor dental hygiene, are at an increased risk of intraoral cancer. Carcinomas of the lip are related to sunlight exposure.

Anatomy

The oral cavity consists of the lip, floor of mouth, oral tongue (anterior two-thirds), buccal mucosa, upper and lower gingiva, hard palate, and retromolar trigone.

The mylohyoid muscle forms the floor of the oral cavity. The roof of the oral cavity is the hard palate. Anteriorly the oral cavity extends to the skin-vermillion junction. Posteriorly, the oral cavity extends to the retromolar trigone (which is a triangular area of mucosa which covers the mandible, posterior to the last molar tooth), and the posterior oral tongue, which is separated from the base of the tongue by the circumvallate papillae.

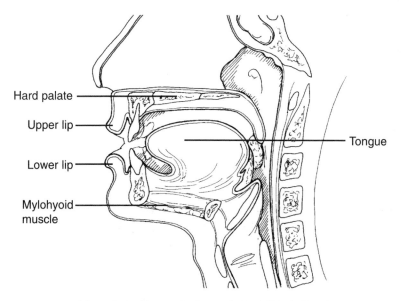

Fig. 1.6 Boundaries of the Oral Cavity

CARCINOMA OF THE LIP

Routes of Spread

Squamous cell carcinomas of the lip most commonly arise from the lower lip and spread by direct invasion. Lip carcinomas present with lymph node metastases 5-10% of the time. The lip drains to lymph nodes in the submental, sub-maxillary and jugulodigastric regions. Lymph node involve-ment increases with large lesions, poorly differentiated tumors, spread to the wet mucosal surfaces, invasion of the dermis, or recurrent disease.

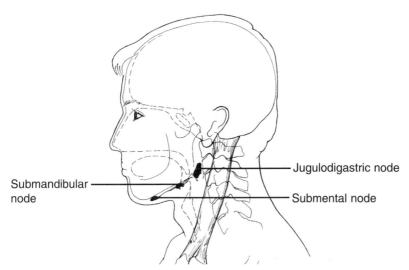

Fig. 1.7 Lymph Drainage of the Lip

Treatment

Carcinoma in-situ and early lesions of the lip (less than 0.5-1.5 cm) may be treated with surgical excision alone. Radiation therapy is used for commissure lesions, or lesions that would create a large surgical or functional defect (upper lip lesion or greater than 1.5 cm of the lower lip). Advanced lesions with bone or neural invasion require resection and postoperative radiation.

Technical Aspects of Radiation Therapy

The radiation portal should include the primary lesion with a 2 cm margin. A shield made of lead and a bolus material to absorb backscatter, should be placed under the lip to block the alveolar process and gums. Elective neck treatment may be withheld since neck failures from lip cancers have proven to be salvageable.

Dose

Lip treatment can be given with superficial or orthovoltage x-rays, electrons, or with brachytherapy.
External beam doses: 60-70 Gy at 2.0 Gy per fraction, depending on the size of the lesion and method of treatment.

FLOOR OF MOUTH AND ORAL TONGUE

Routes of Spread

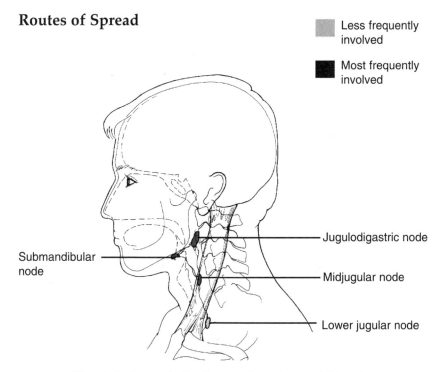

Fig. 1.8 Lymph Drainage for Floor of Mouth

Floor of mouth and oral tongue lesions more commonly present with lymph node metastases with an incidence of 35-40%. The primary nodal drainage is to the jugulodigastric, midjugular, and submaxillary lymph nodes. These are usually midline tumors and therefore bilateral lymph node chains are at risk for disease. These tumors may infiltrate locally to involve underlying muscle, or extend along fibrofatty planes.

Treatment

Surgery and radiation therapy both have similar cure rates for T1 and T2 (4 cm or less) cancers of the floor of mouth and oral tongue.

Treatment is generally given by external beam which provides treatment to the primary lesion and neck nodes. The intraoral cone or an interstitial implant can be used for small cancers, as definitive treatment or as a boost. The advantage of using the intraoral cone or an interstitial implant is sparing the normal tissues that would otherwise be included in the external beam portal. If the intraoral cone is used in conjunction with external beam, the cone field should be treated before the large lateral fields so that the patient can tolerate manipulation of the mouth before mucositis begins.

Surgery with postoperative radiation is advocated for T3 or T4 tumors (greater than 4 cm or with invasion of adjacent structures), close or positive margins, perineural or lymphatic vascular invasion, or multiple positive nodes.

Technical Aspects of Radiation Therapy

The borders for the lateral fields for floor of mouth or oral tongue include:

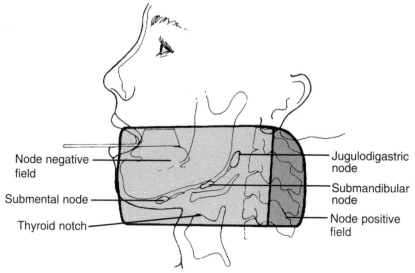

Fig. 1.9 Treatment Field for Floor of Mouth/Oral Tongue Tumor

A tongue blade is used to raise the roof of the mouth out of the treatment field.

Anterior - in front of the mandible (exclude the lower lip if possible)

Posterior - *node negative* -behind vertebral bodies
node positive -behind spinous processes

Superior - 1.5 cm above the tongue

Inferior - thyroid notch

NOTE: In patients with well-lateralized lesions and clinically negative neck nodes, an ipsilateral anterior neck field is treated. Bilateral neck nodes must be treated for midline tumors, or with patients with positive nodes.

Dose

Floor of mouth and oral tongue tumors are treated postoperatively to 50 Gy at 1.8 Gy per fraction (off cord at 45 Gy), with a boost to 60 Gy for negative margins, 65 Gy for positive margins, and to 70 Gy for gross disease.

An intraoral cone, using electrons (usually 9-12 MeV), or orthovoltage, can be used for a boost. Bolus may be utilized, depending on the depth of the lesion. Generally, for a boost 15-24 Gy is given at 2-2.75 Gy per fraction.

After the introral cone boost or implant, external beam radiation is delivered to all nodal areas that are potentially involved with microscopic disease to at least 50 Gy (see the dose section in Treatment of the Neck).

OROPHARYNX

Carcinomas of the oropharynx are relatively rare head and neck cancers. 95% of oropharyngeal lesions are squamous cell carcinomas. Lymphomas and lymphoepithelial tumors are rare but can occur in the tonsil and in the base of the tongue. Risk factors include smoking, alcohol consumption, and poor dental hygiene.

Anatomy

The oropharynx includes the base of the tongue, the tonsillar region, (the vallecula is considered part of the tonsillar fossa and pillars), the soft palate, and the portion of the pharyngeal wall between the pharyngoepiglottic fold and the nasopharynx. The oropharynx is bound anteriorly by the circumvallate papillae, and the junction of the hard and soft palate. The oropharynx extends from the highest aspect of the soft palate superiorly to the hyoid bone inferiorly and is bound posteriorly by the posterior pharyngeal wall.

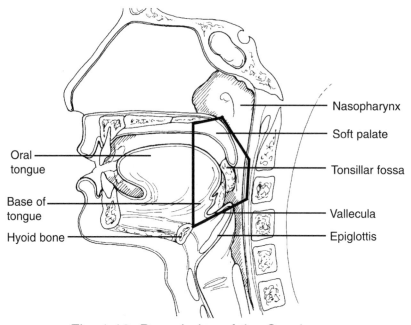

Fig. 1.10 Boundaries of the Orophayrnx

Routes of Spread

Oropharyngeal tumors spread primarily by direct extension or through the lymphatics. Hematogenous spread can occur with advanced or recurrent tumors. The most common site of hematogenous metastases is the lungs.

The first echelon of lymph node drainage of the oropharyngeal region is to the jugulodigastric and midjugular nodes. The incidence of lymph node involvement, and the risk of bilateral disease, or positive cervical nodes, depends on the location and the size of the primary tumor.

14

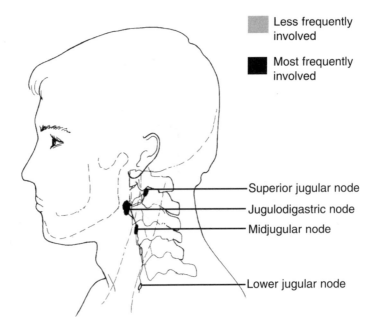

Fig 1.11 Lymph Drainage of the Oropharynx

Technical Aspects of Radiation Therapy

Radiation therapy is the treatment of choice for early stage oropharyngeal tumors. Large extensive tumors are treated with combined surgery and postoperative radiation. Radiation therapy alone is often used for inoperable patients and for palliation.

Lateral parallel opposed fields for tumors of the oropharynx:

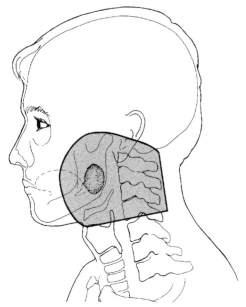

Fig. 1.12 Lateral Treatment Field for Oropharynx Tumor

Anterior - 2 cm anterior to the tumor
Posterior - behind the spinous process (to include the posterior cervical lymph nodes)
Superior - entire jugular chain and above C1 (to include the retropharyngeal lymph nodes)
Inferior - thyroid notch

An anterior lower neck field is used to treat supraclavicular and lower jugular lymph nodes. Treatment of the lower neck is essential because of the high rate of bilateral lymph node metastases even if the neck is clinically negative. Tonsillar lesions which are lateralized may only need ipsilateral neck node treatment.

For tumors of the base of tongue, the final boost field may be administered by interstitial implant (for small anterior-lateral lesions), a submental external beam portal, or a reduced lateral field.

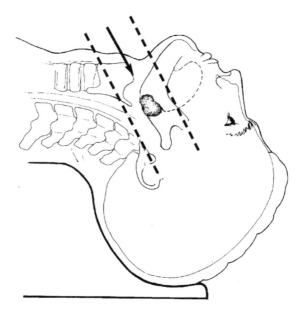

Fig. 1.13   Boost Field for Tumors of the Base of Tongue

The submental technique has the advantage of limiting the dose to the mandible. Tumor extension to the oral tongue however, would be a contraindication for this method. (The oral tongue would be too deep when boosting from the submental approach and would receive a poor dose distribution).

Postoperative treatment is advocated with close or positive margins, multiple positive lymph nodes, extracapsular extension, or elective neck coverage.

Dose

Doses of 50 Gy at 1.8 Gy per fraction (off cord at 45 Gy) are advocated with boosts to 70-75 Gy for primary oropharyngeal tumors. Postoperative total doses vary, but range from 50-70 Gy, depending upon the pathological findings and the extent of the tumor at the time of surgery.

Hyperfractionation may be used for advanced tumors, for a total dose of 74.4 Gy at 1.2 Gy per fraction, twice a day, with a 6 hour interval in between. The port should be reduced off cord at 45 Gy, and can be reduced again at 50 Gy.

LARYNX

Carcinoma of the larynx is the most common cancer of the head and neck. 65% of laryngeal carcinomas occur in the glottic larynx and 34% occur in the supraglottic larynx. Subglottic carcinomas are rare, comprising only 1% of all glottic cancers.

Laryngeal cancers are more common in men than in women, with a ratio of 5:1. Cigarette smoking is a known etiologic factor for laryngeal cancer. The most common histology is squamous cell. Patients with vocal cord carcinoma commonly present with hoarseness, while supraglottic tumors can cause sore throat and odynophagia.

Anatomy

The larynx is subdivided into three regions: the supraglottis, the glottis, and the subglottis. The supraglottic larynx is the largest region and consists of the laryngeal surface of the epiglottis, the aryepiglottic folds, the arytenoids, the false vocal cords and the laryngeal ventricles.

The structures of the glottis include: the right and left true vocal cords, and the anterior and posterior commissures. The majority of glottic lesions arise from the anterior one-half of the vocal cords. The anterior commissure is usually within 1.0 cm from the skin surface. Because of this location, special attention must be given to the anterior border when designing the treatment portal for glottic cancers.

The subglottis extends from 0.5 cm below the glottis to the lower margin of the cricoid cartilage and is generally 1.5 cm in length.

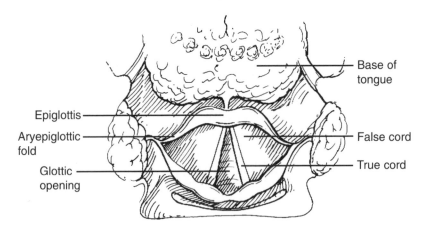

Fig. 1.14 The Larynx (Superior View)

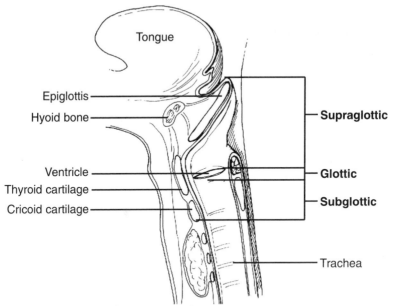

Fig. 1.15 Subdivisions of the Larynx (Left Lateral View)

Routes of Spread

There are no capillary lymphatics in the true vocal cords. Therefore, lymph node metastases do not occur until the tumor spreads beyond the true vocal cords. The incidence of lymph node metastases for a tumor confined to the true vocal cords is 0-2%. For advanced disease the incidence increases to 10-20%. Tumors of the supraglottic larynx present with lymph node metastases 55% of the time, with the first echelon of nodal drainage being the jugulodigastric and the midjugular lymph nodes.

Glottic tumors often spread by local invasion to the supraglottic or subglottic regions. Impairment in the mobility of the vocal cords may occur by direct invasion of the tumor into the underlying intrinsic muscle (thyroarytenoid). Vocal cord immobility is a poor prognostic indicator. The incidence of distant metastases is 10-20% with the lung being the most common site for metastatic disease.

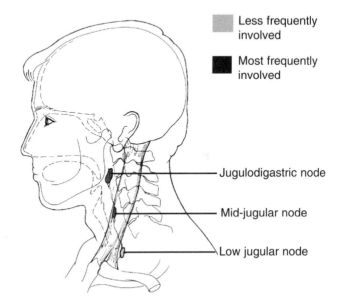

Fig. 1.16 Lymph Drainage of the Larynx

Treatment of Glottic Cancer

The goal of therapy for laryngeal cancer is curative treatment with minimal functional impairment. Treatment options for early glottic lesions include external beam radiation, hemi-laryngectomy, cordectomy or transoral removal of the lesion. Radiation therapy is the preferred treatment in early stage tumors to preserve voice quality with excellent cure rates. Surgery is generally reserved for salvage.

Technical Aspects of Radiation Therapy

For a T1 lesion (confined to the vocal cord), the portal is limited to the vocal cords. The lymphatics are not electively treated since the risk of involvement is only 0-2%.

The glottic larynx is treated through parallel opposed lateral fields. The borders, which can be clinically palpated, are described below:

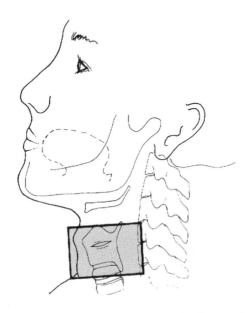

Fig. 1.17 Treatment Port for Early Stage Larynx

Anterior - 1.5-2 cm beyond the thyroid cartilage
Superior - top of thyroid cartilage
Posterior - anterior margin of the vertebral bodies
Inferior -   below the cricoid cartilage

For T2 lesions, with normal cord mobility and minimal tumor extension, treatment portals are designed with a 2-3 cm margin around the tumor. Depending on the extent of the lesion, the jugulodigastric and midjugular nodes may be covered in the treatment port, especially in patients with impaired cord mobility.

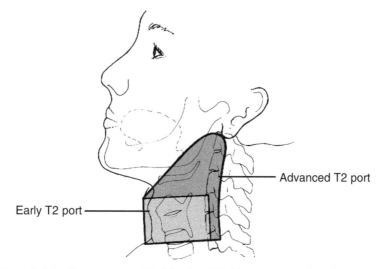

Fig. 1.18 Treatment Fields for T2 Tumors of the Larynx

Superior - supraglottic extension and 2-3 cm margin
Anterior - 1.5-2 cm beyond the thyroid cartilage
Posterior - mid-vertebral bodies
Inferior - infraglottic extension and 2-3 cm margin

Advanced or bulky lesions of the glottic larynx (T3 and T4: cord fixation, destruction of cartilage, or extension beyond the larynx) are best treated with total laryngectomy. Post-operative radiation is administered if indicated.

Patients on protocol are presently undergoing trials of chemotherapy and radiation versus radiation alone for patients with fixed vocal cords (T3). Radiation may also be used for palliation in inoperable patients.

Lateral parallel opposed fields for T3 or T4 or node positive patients:

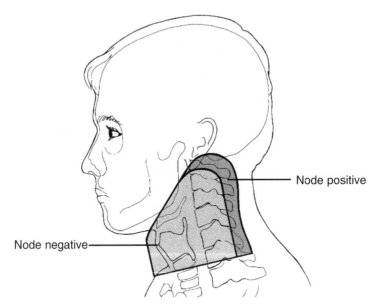

Fig. 1.19 Lateral Port for T3/T4 or Node Positive Larynx

Anterior - 1.5-2 cm beyond the thyroid cartilage
Posterior - *node negative* - behind the mastoid process to
include the midjugular nodes
node positive - behind the spinous process to
include the posterior cervical lymph nodes
Superior - *node negative* - 2 cm above the angle of the
mandible to treat the jugulodigastric nodes
node positive - above the mastoid process to
cover the entire jugulodigastric lymph node
chain. (The hyoid bone and epiglottis are included to incorporate the pre-epiglottic space)
Inferior - below the cricoid cartilage

An anterior lower neck portal should be added to treat the
supraclavicular and lower jugular lymph nodes (see
Treatment of the Neck section).

Treatment of Supraglottic Larynx

Early supraglottic carcinomas are best managed by external beam radiation or supraglottic laryngectomy. For early tumors with minimal local extension and normal cord mobility, radiation is advocated.

Bulky, advanced lesions, that have fixed cords, or cartilage invasion can be managed with total laryngectomy and radical neck dissection. Postoperative radiation is delivered when indicated. Advanced disease may be treated with chemotherapy and radiation versus radiation alone on protocol. Radiation may also be used for palliation in inoperable patients.

Lateral parallel opposed portal for supraglottic tumors:

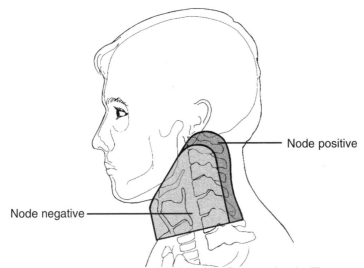

Fig. 1.20 Treatment Fields for Supraglottic Tumors

Anterior - 1.5-2 cm beyond the thyroid cartilage
Posterior -*node negative* - behind the mastoid process to
            include the midjugular nodes

node positive - behind the spinous process to include the posterior cervical lymph nodes

Superior - *node negative* - 2 cm above the angle of the mandible to treat the jugulodigastric nodes
node positive - above the mastoid process to treat the entire jugulodigastric lymph node chain (the hyoid bone and epiglottis are included to incorporate the pre-epiglottic space)

Inferior - bottom of the cricoid cartilage and 2 cm below the lowest extent of disease.

A boost portal should be designed to encompass the involved lymph nodes, and the primary tumor with a 1 cm margin.

An anterior neck field is added for T2, T3 and T4 disease. The tracheal stoma should be electively treated in the anterior neck field in patients who have an emergency tracheotomy, or who exhibit subglottic extension, close or positive tracheal margin, or involvement of the soft tissues of the neck (See Treatment of the Neck section).

Dose

Linear accelerators of 4 mV or Co-60 machines are most commonly used. Because of the skin-sparing effect of higher energies, bolus may be needed with energies of 6 mV. Wedges are used with lateral neck fields to compensate for the contour.

Glottic

Glottic lesions that are confined to the vocal cords (T1) are standardly treated to 66 Gy at 2.0 Gy per fraction.

Lesions with supraglottic or subglottic extension (T2) may

be treated with conventional fractionation with doses of 66-70 Gy at 2.0 Gy per fraction. More advanced tumors require boosts to 70-75 Gy.

Lesions with extension beyond the vocal cords (T2-T4) may be hyperfractionated to a total dose of 74.4-76.8 Gy at 1.2 Gy twice a day, with a 6 hour interval in between.

In either case, lateral fields are reduced off the spinal cord after 45 Gy. The posterior neck nodes may be boosted with electrons. An anterior neck field is used to treat extensive lesions (T3-T4) and node positive patients.

Supraglottic

For T1 tumors (confined to one subsite) the total dose is generally 66 Gy at 2.0 Gy per fraction to the lateral boost fields. The spinal cord should be excluded from the lateral field after 45 Gy. More advanced tumors require boosts to 70-75 Gy.

For patients with advanced disease, who are treated primarily with radiation, hyperfractionation can be used to total doses of 74.4 Gy-76.8 Gy at 1.2 Gy per fraction twice a day. The initial lateral fields are treated to 50.4 Gy. The spinal cord is excluded after 45 Gy. The posterior neck nodes may be boosted with electrons after the spinal cord is blocked. Postoperative total doses vary, but range from 50-70 Gy, depending upon the pathological findings and the extent of the tumor at the time of surgery. An anterior neck field is used to treat extensive lesions and node positive patients.

HYPOPHARYNX

The most common site for presentation of hypopharyngeal tumors is in the pyriform sinus, followed by the posterior pharyngeal wall. Postcricoid tumors are rare. 95% of hypopharyngeal tumors are squamous cell. These tumors are seen more frequently in men than women and are associated with alcohol and tobacco abuse. Patients often present with either a localized sore throat, a neck mass, dysphagia or ear pain.

Anatomy

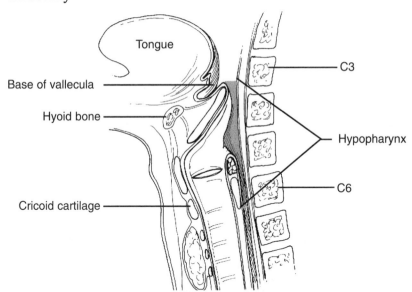

Fig. 1.21   Boundaries of the Hypopharynx

The hypopharynx includes the pyriform sinus, postcricoid area, and the posterior pharyngeal wall.

The superior border of the hypopharynx is the pharyngoepiglottic fold and the base of the vallecula which is located radiographically at the level of the hyoid bone.

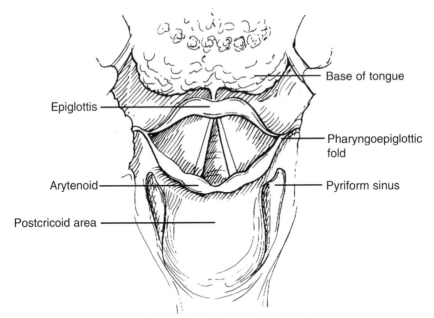

Fig. 1.21   Posterior View of Hypopharynx

The inferior border is the beginning of the esophagus which is at the lower border of the cricoid cartilage. The pyriform sinus has three walls and opens into the hypopharynx posteriorly.

Routes of Spread

The hypopharynx has a rich lymphatic supply. About 75% of pyriform sinus tumors, 60% of posterior pharyngeal wall tumors, and 40% of postcricoid tumors will present with lymph node metastases. The jugulodigastric and midjugular lymph nodes are most commonly involved as well as the parapharyngeal lymph nodes. Also, tumors may metastasize to the posterior cervical chain. At presentation, 20-30% of patients have distant metastases, with the lung being the most common site. Hypopharyngeal tumors also spread by local invasion.

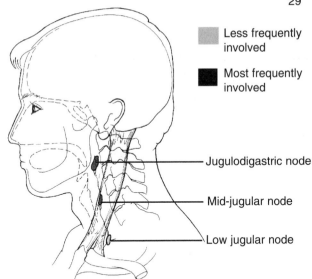

Fig. 1.22 Lymph Drainage of the Hypopharynx

Treatment

Radiation therapy alone is preferred for early lesions of the hypopharynx (with normal vocal cord mobility and without bone invasion) with excellent local control. With radiation therapy, swallowing and speech may be preserved and bilateral coverage of the neck can be accomplished. Bulky tumors that have laryngeal or cartilage involvement or extend into the soft tissues of the neck should be treated with combined surgery and postoperative radiation therapy if possible. Tumors with apex involvement often have cartilage invasion. Medically inoperable patients and unresectable lesions should be treated with radiation.

Early lesions of the pharyngeal wall may be treated with radiation therapy alone. It is controversial whether the larger lesions should be treated with radiation alone versus resection and postoperative radiation.

The optimal treatment for postcricoid lesions is presently undefined. In general, if these lesions can be resected, postoperative radiation is given. For unresectable lesions, radiation is used alone.

Technical Aspects of Radiation Therapy

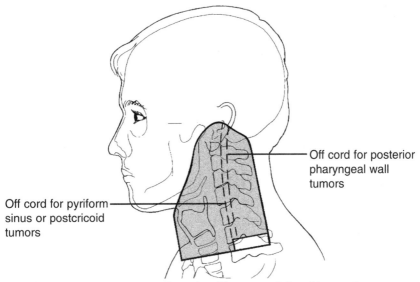

Off cord for posterior pharyngeal wall tumors

Off cord for pyriform sinus or postcricoid tumors

Fig. 1.23 Treatment Port for Tumor of the Hypopharynx

Superior - inferior border of mandible and mastoid process (include margin on the jugulodigastric node which is located at the angle of the mandible), to the base of the skull (to cover the retropharyngeal nodes and the entire jugular chain lymph nodes).

Anterior - in front of the thyroid cartilage with a margin around tumor extension

Posterior -behind the spinous processes with a margin on all nodal disease (to include the posterior cervical lymph nodes)

Inferior - below the cricoid cartilage, to encompass the entire extent of the tumor with a 1.5-2 cm margin

An anterior neck field is added to treat the supraclavicular nodes. For postoperative treatment, the spinal cord block should be placed in the lateral field so that the stoma may receive an adequate dose.

Dose

Postoperative - 50 Gy to large fields at 1.8-2.0 Gy per fraction. Block the entire spinal cord at 45 Gy. The initial area of gross disease is boosted to 60 Gy for negative margins, 66 Gy for positive margins, and 70 Gy for gross disease.

When treating with definitive radiation therapy, boost doses to 66-70 Gy may be used, depending on the stage of the tumor.

Currently, hyperfractionated schedules are being used with excellent results. Patients are treated to doses of 50 Gy at 1.2 Gy per fraction, twice a day. The spinal cord is blocked at 45 Gy, and gross disease plus a margin, is boosted to 74.4 Gy.

Negative posterior neck nodes are boosted with electrons to 50 Gy. If the neck nodes are positive then the nodes are boosted to at least 60 Gy. Higher doses may be used for gross nodal disease.

In all of the above treatment schemes, a separate anterior neck field is used to treat the lower jugular and supraclavicular lymph nodes (see the section on Treatment of the Neck).

NASOPHARYNX

Although tumors of the nasopharynx are common in southern China, they are relatively rare in the United States. 85-90% of all nasopharyngeal tumors are epidermoid or undifferentiated carcinomas. Lymphomas comprise the remaining 10-15%.

Anatomy

The nasopharynx is a cuboidal structure with a rich lymphatic supply. It is bordered by the sphenoid sinus superiorly, the clivus and the first two cervical vertebrae posteriorly, the soft palate inferiorly, and the posterior choanae anteriorly.

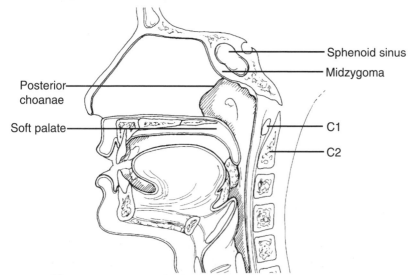

Fig. 1.24   Boundaries of the Nasopharynx

An external landmark denoting the roof of the nasopharynx (or the floor of the sphenoid sinus) is the mid-zygoma which is a point midway between the external auditory canal and the lateral canthus.

Routes of Spread

80-90% of nasopharyngeal cancers present with positive cervical nodes and approximately 50% of these will have bilateral nodal disease. There is no correlation between the size of the primary and the degree of lymph node involvement or the rate of distant metastasis. Nasopharyngeal tumors can also spread by direct extension. The sites for direct extension of the tumor include the tumor growing through the soft palate, into the nasal cavity, or through the base of the skull. Generally, the foramen lacerum is the opening through which nasopharyngeal tumors extend into the middle cranial fossa.

Lymphatic drainage of the nasopharynx is by three major routes:

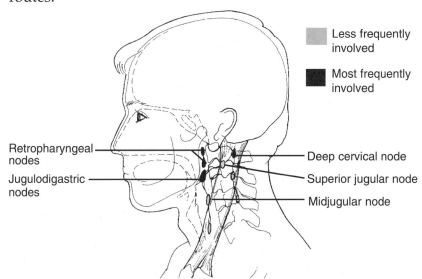

Fig. 1.25   Lymph Drainage of the Nasopharynx

1) the retropharyngeal nodes (retroparotid) - the upper most node in this group is the node of Rouviere. These nodes lie anterior to C1 and C2 vertebral bodies.

34

2) the deep cervical nodes (junctional nodes) which lie behind the sternocleidomastoid muscle at the junction of the spinal accessory nodes and jugular nodes.
3) the jugulodiagastric node

Technical Aspects of Radiation Therapy

Surgical resection of tumors of the nasopharynx is not possible; therefore, radiation therapy is recommended as definitive treatment.

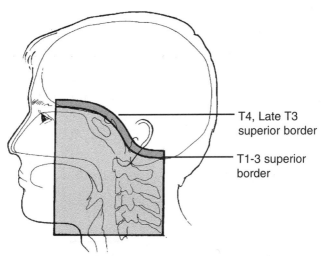

Fig. 1.26 Treatment Volumes for Nasopharynx Tumors

The treatment volume for T1, T2, and T3 lesions (i.e., no base of skull or cranial nerve involvement) should include:

Anterior - posterior 2 cm of nasal cavity (or 2 cm beyond tumor extension). Posterior 1/3 of the maxillary sinus, posterior ethmoid sinuses, and the posterior 1/4 of the orbit

Superior -entire sphenoid sinus, cavernous sinus, base of skull (with at least a 0.5 cm margin)

Posterior -Behind spinous processes to include retropharyngeal nodes, posterior pharyngeal wall, deep cervical nodes, or posterior cervical nodes.

In addition to the lateral neck fields described above, an anterior neck field to include the supraclavicular and lower cervical nodes, should be treated because of the high probability of nodal spread.

For T4 tumors, the margins of the lateral treatment field should include the pituitary, and encompass all intracranial extension.

Dose

Typically, 50.4 Gy at 1.8 Gy/day (or at 1.2 Gy treating twice a day for T2-T4 lesions) is given to the initial lateral neck target volume, reducing the port off of the spinal cord at 45 Gy. A boost field is then given to the nasopharynx and nodal disease to 65 Gy for T1-T2 and 70-75 Gy for T3-T4 tumors. Lymphoepitheliomas are a histologic type of nasopharyngeal tumors that are more radiosensitive than squamous cell. For this histopathologic type of tumors, the total dose is decreased approximately 4-5 Gy for the respective stages.

The anterior neck field is generally treated to a total dose of 45-50 Gy at 1.8 Gy/day.

MAXILLARY SINUS

Of the paranasal sinuses, the maxillary sinus is most frequently involved with carcinoma. Histopathologically, 80%
of maxillary sinus tumors are squamous cell, 15% are adenocarcinomas, and the remaining 5% are lymphomas,
melanomas, or sarcomas. These tumors usually do not pro-
duce symptoms until they extend beyond the sinus walls.

Anatomy

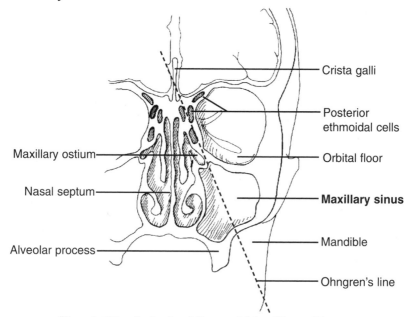

Fig. 1.27   Anterior View of Maxillary Sinus

The maxillary sinus is bound by the following structures:
Superior wall - floor of orbit
Medial wall -   thin walls of the nasal fossa
Inferior wall -   alveolar process and hard palate
Posterior wall - posterior wall of the maxillary which sepa-
                   rates the sinus from the pterygopalatine
                   fossa and infratemporal fossa.

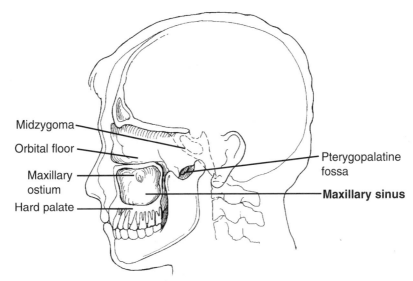

Fig. 1.28   The Maxillary Sinus (Lateral View)

Note that the floor of the maxillary sinus extends inferior to the floor of the nasal cavity and the roof is superior to the infraorbital rim. Also note the proximity of the posterior wall to the nasopharynx and the pterygopalatine fossa. These anatomic landmarks will be important for treatment set-up.

Routes of Spread

Tumors of the maxillary sinus are usually advanced at presentation with local invasion of bone. Tumors may present with:

medial extension - through the nasal fossa, ethmoid or frontal sinus (the maxillary ostium is a pathway for medial extension). Patients with gross disease in the ethmoid sinus should be considered to have microscopic orbital extension.

inferior extension -through the hard palate

posterior extension - into the pterygopalatine fossa or the
base of the skull
superior extension - through the floor of the orbit
anterior or lateral extension - through the walls of the
maxillary sinus to the cheek.

Lymphatic spread from early carcinomas of the maxillary
sinus is rare. Once the tumor has extended beyond the bony
walls of the maxillary sinus the tumor is able to reach a
richer capillary and lymphatic supply. Overall, 8-15% of
maxillary sinus tumors present with lymphatic spread. The
pathways of lymphatic drainage depend on the area of
invasion. Lesions that invade the oral cavity and cheek
drain to the submandibular and upper jugular lymph
nodes. Tumors that invade through the nasal fossa and
nasopharynx drain to the retropharyngeal and superior
jugular lymph nodes.

Treatment

Initial surgical resection is recommended when possible.
Early infrastructure lesions may be treated with surgery
alone. Postoperative radiation therapy is generally recommended for all other patients. Patients who present with
invasion through the posterior wall of the maxillary sinus
(invasion of the nasopharynx and/or base of the skull) are
generally inoperable and must be treated with radiation
alone.

Technical Aspects of Radiation Therapy

Treatment set up is by an anterior and either one or two lateral wedged fields. The three field technique with two lateral fields is recommended for deep medial lesions. A tongue
blade is used to displace the tongue inferiorly from the
treatment field.

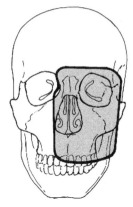
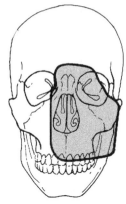
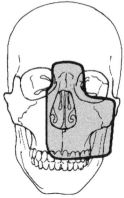

Fig. 1.29a
Orbital Involvement

Fig. 1.29b
Lacrimal Gland Block

Fig. 1.29c
No Orbital Involvement

Anterior field borders:
The superior and lateral aspects of the field depend on the extent of orbital involvement.

Superior - 2 cm above the cribiform plate (to cover the ethmoid sinuses)

> _no orbital involvement_: include the floor of the ipsilateral orbit but remain below the cornea (Remember: the floor of the maxillary sinus slopes upward). The patient should look straight ahead to avoid overdosage to the retina.
> _orbital involvement_: treat the entire orbit (with an adequate margin around the tumor). Depending on the extent of orbital involvement, the lacrimal gland may be shielded at 40 Gy (unless the shielding compromises the dose to the initial gross tumor volume).

Inferior - lateral commissure of the lip (this will provide a margin on the lower border of the maxillary sinus) to include the alveolar ridge.

Medial - 1.5-2 cm across the midline to include the ethmoid sinus and the medial aspect of the contralateral orbit

Lateral - to include the entire maxillary sinus tumor extent with an adequate margin (if the infratemporal fossa is involved, fall off is needed laterally)

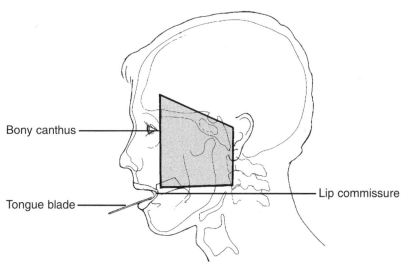

Bony canthus

Lip commissure

Tongue blade

Fig. 1.30   Lateral Treatment Field of Maxillary Sinus Tumor

Lateral field borders:

Anterior - behind the contralateral bony canthus (the lateral portals can be angled 5 degrees posteriorly to shield the contralateral lens)

Superior - 2 cm above the cribiform plate and follow the floor of the cranium with a margin on the clivus

Posterior- include the pterygopalatine fossa and the nasopharynx with a margin on the posterior extent of the tumor. In patients with nasal cavity/nasopharynx involvement, include the retropharyngeal nodes. This border usually bisects the vertebral bodies. If possible, do not overlap the spinal cord because it will also receive dose from the anterior field. With posterior tumors the spinal cord must be included, and it is imperative that careful dosimetry be done for cord tolerance.

Inferior - lateral commissure of the lip

Tissue tolerance of critical structures such as the contralateral optic nerve, and optic chiasm, lacrimal apparatus, spinal cord and retina necessitate tailored, planned field reductions.

Neck nodes are not routinely treated but should be included in patients with recurrent tumors, extension into the oral cavity, oropharynx, nasopharynx, or positive neck nodes. If the patient has had a lymph node dissection, the neck should be treated for multiple positive nodes or extracapsular extension. Bilateral lymph nodes are treated since the areas of invasion (oral cavity, oropharynx, and nasopharynx) are midline structures.

Dose

The maxillary sinus fields are treated to 50 Gy at 1.8-2.0 Gy per fraction. The initial area of gross disease is boosted to 60 Gy for negative margins, and 65 Gy for positive margins. When treating with definitive radiation therapy boost doses may total 66-70 Gy, depending on the tumor volume. Bolus should be placed on any gross disease or subcutaneous skin involvement. Bolus can also be used on a large surgical defect to increase homogeneity. Wedges are frequently used and the fields are weighted for homogeneity.

PAROTID

The parotid gland is the largest of the salivary glands. The majority of all salivary gland tumors, both benign and malignant, occur in this gland. The word parotid means "around the ear".

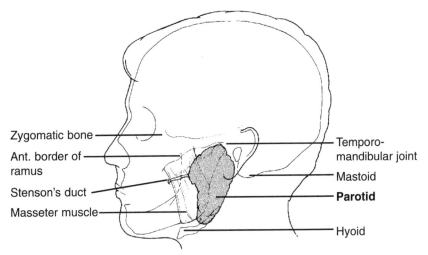

Fig. 1.31 Boundaries of the Parotid Gland

Anatomy

The parotid gland is shaped by the structures which surround it. The superior border lies below the zygomatic arch, and below and in front of the external auditory meatus. Posteriorly, it extends to the tip of the mastoid. Anteriorly, the gland extends as far as the orifice of the parotid duct (Stenson's duct), which is adjacent to the second molar tooth. Inferiorly, the gland extends to the upper border of the posterior belly of the digastric muscle, which radiographically lies between the mandible and the hyoid bone. The facial nerve artificially divides the parotid gland into superficial and deep lobes. The parotid gland contains

nodes within the substance of the gland and the first echelon of drainage is to the ipsilateral jugulodiagastric lymph
node.

Routes of Spread

The superficial lymph nodes of the parotid receive drainage
from the skin, subcutaneous tissue of the face, auricle, middle ear, and external auditory canal. Due to this drainage,
the parotid is commonly involved with metastatic disease
as well as primary parotid tumors. Most malignant tumors
spread through local invasion, ipsilateral neck lymph node
spread, and perineural invasion. 25% of parotid tumors present with lymph node metastases and 25% have facial nerve
palsy from the invasion of cranial nerve VII.

Technical Aspects of Radiation Therapy

The primary treatment for parotid tumors is surgery.
Radiation therapy is indicated for: 1) high grade tumors,
2) positive margins, 3) perineural involvement, 4) positive
neck nodes, or 5) recurrent disease.

The treatment volume includes the parotid bed and the ipsilateral upper neck nodes. For high grade lesions or positive
nodes, the ipsilateral lower neck may be treated. If the
tumor shows perineural invasion, the base of the skull
should be included to cover the cranial nerve pathway.

44

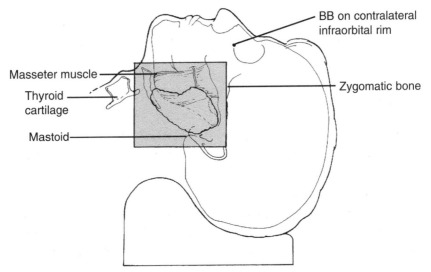

Fig. 1.32 Treatment Port for Parotid Tumor

Superior border - zygomatic arch (including all of surgical scar)
Anterior border - anterior border of masseter muscle
Posterior border -behind mastoid process
Inferior border - Top of thyroid cartilage

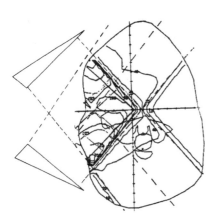

Fig. 1. Oblique Paired Wedge Field for Parotid Tumor

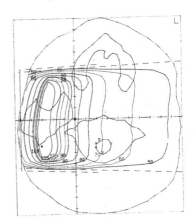

Fig. 1. Lateral Mixed Beam Field

The parotid bed can be treated through either an oblique paired wedge field, or by using mixed beams from a lateral field. When using a paired wedge field, special attention should be given to make sure that the lower bony orbit is above the superior border of the exit of the posterior oblique field, and that only the anterior wedged field over-lies the spinal cord.

Dose

Parotid lesions which have been completely resected should be treated to a total dose of 55-60 Gy (1.8-2.0 Gy/day) at a depth of 5 cm or to the deepest extent of the parotid on pre-operative CT scan. Lesions which were not completely resected should be boosted to 65 Gy.

Chapter 2

Central Nervous System Tumors

HIGH GRADE GLIOMAS

Primary tumors of the brain represent less than 2% of all malignancies in the United States. Astrocytomas account for 50% of all primary central nervous system tumors. Astrocytomas can be divided into three categories: well-differentiated (mild hypercellularity and pleomorphism), anaplastic (increased pleomorphism and proliferative activity) and glioblastoma multiforme (tumor necrosis is present). High grade astrocytomas (anaplastic astrocytomas and glioblastoma multiforme) primarily occur in the elderly population, 50-80 year old. Overall the five year survival is less than 10%.

Anatomy

The central nervous system is composed of gray and white matter. Gray matter is made of oligodendroglia, astrocytes, and non-dividing neurons. White matter is composed of nerve fibers, axons, oligodendroglia, and supporting astrocytes. Astrocytomas predominately arise in the white matter. These tumors tend to present as a single mass arising in one hemisphere. Astrocytomas in adults most commonly arise in the cerebrum. 75% of astrocytomas are supratentorial. The cerebellum is the most common infratentorial site, and these tumors are more commonly seen in the younger age group.

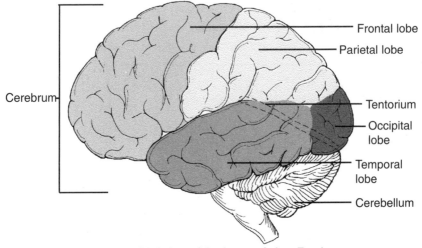

Fig. 2.1 Divisional Lobes of the Brain

Routes of Spread

Gliomas primarily spread through local invasion along the pre-existing pathways defined by white matter tracts. The extent of infiltration may be a long distance from the primary tumor. Tumor cells have been found on biopsy series in the peritumoral edema. Anaplastic astrocytomas and glioblastoma multiforme may also seed the cerebrospinal fluid.

Treatment

For high grade astrocytomas, radiation therapy is delivered after biopsy or resection. Whole brain irradiation was advocated in the past due to both the infiltrative nature of these tumors and the fact that CT and MRI were not available for imaging. Since the development of CT and MRI, limited radiation fields encompassing the contrast enhanced lesion with a margin, have been advocated. Even though spinal seeding is a mode of spread, craniospinal irradiation is not advocated since local failure is the predominate problem. Limited field irradiation provides equal (although poor) survival rates compared to whole brain irradiation. With limited fields there is less damage to the central nervous system in the few long term survivors. Whole brain irradiation is reserved for multifocal lesions, or lesions with ependymal involvement.

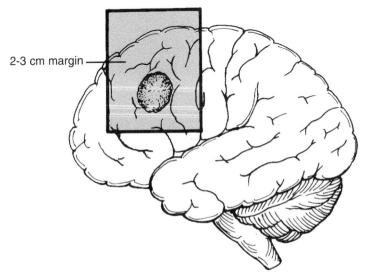

2-3 cm margin

Fig. 2.2 Lateral Treament Port for Glioma

Technical Aspects of Radiation Therapy

A 2-3 cm margin is generally placed around the contrast enhanced tumor volume and surrounding edema, using preoperative scans. Adequate coverage of the tumor volume may be accomplished with two or more treatment fields. Two fields, in a wedged pair arrangement, may offer sparing of the opposite cortex.

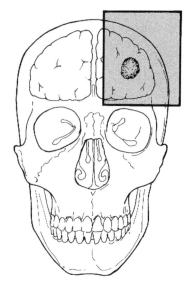

Fig. 2.3   Anterior Treatment Field for Glioma

Dose

Conventional radiation therapy doses for partial brain fields are standardly 60 Gy at 1.8-2.0 Gy per fraction. The portal may be reduced after 50 Gy, if the initial portal is large. The reduced portal should encompass the contrast enhanced tumor, not including edema, with a 2-3 cm margin,

PITUITARY TUMORS

About 10% of all symptomatic intracranial tumors arise in the pituitary gland. Asymptomatic adenomas are found 10-20% of the time at autopsy. Patients with pituitary adenomas may present with endocrine abnormalities as a result of hypersecretion of hormones caused by the tumor. Visual impairment, due to encroachment of the tumor on the optic chiasm, is another common presentation. Patients with large adenomas may also present with cranial nerve abnormalities due to encroachment on the cranial nerves which lie lateral to the sella turcica in the cavernous sinus.

There are three histological subtypes of pituitary tumors. The chromophobe adenomas, which are endocrine inactive, are the most common. Acidophillic adenomas may secrete growth hormone or prolactin. The third type, basophilic adenomas, may secrete ACTH, thyroid stimulating hormone or follicle stimulating hormone.

Anatomy

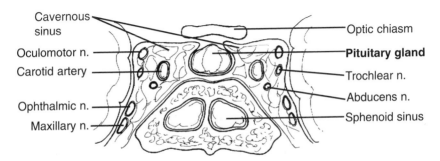

Fig. 2.4 Boundaries of the Pituitary Gland (Frontal Section)

The pituitary gland is a midline structure that lies in the sella turcica. The sella is a saddle-shaped cavity in the body of the sphenoid bone. Radiographically, the sella is located 3/4 inch anterior to, and 3/4 inch above, the external acoustic meatuses. The sphenoid sinus lies below the pituitary. The cavernous sinus is lateral to the pituitary and contains the internal carotid artery and the cranial nerves III, IV, and VI which innervate the eye muscles. This sinus also contains the ophthalmic and maxillary branches of cranial nerve V which supply sensory to the skin of the face. The optic chiasm is usually located anterior and superior to the pituitary.

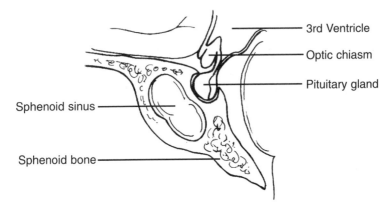

Fig. 2.5 Boundaries of the Pituitary Gland (Sagittal Section)

Routes of Spread

Pituitary adenomas are histologically benign and do not spread through the lymphatics or the bloodstream; however, they can cause damage by local invasion and compression. Tumors which invade laterally into the cavernous sinus may present with extraocular muscle dysfunction from compression of cranial nerves III, IV, and VI. Optic nerve compression may cause bilateral visual loss (bitemporal hemianopsia). Local invasion may also cause headaches, increased intracranial pressure, or cerebrospinal fluid rhinorrhea (from the downward extension of tumor through the sphenoid sinus).

Treatment

Pituitary adenomas are divided into micro- or macroadenomas. Microadenomas are less than 10 mm in size. Microadenomas may be treated with surgery through a transphenoidal resection. Larger tumors may require a craniotomy for removal.

Radiation therapy may be used for definitive treatment or postoperatively. In general, radiation therapy controls hypersecretion in 80% of patients with increased growth hormone, 50-80% with increased ACTH, and 33% with increased secretion of prolactin. However, with radiation, normalization of hormone levels may require months to one year. Patients with a mass effect should undergo surgical decompression to reverse symptoms.

Postoperative radiation is generally recommended after subtotal resection of macroadenomas. It is also recommended after gross total removal of the tumor if there is persistent hormone elevation (consistent with residual disease), or recurrent tumors.

Technical Aspects of Radiation Therapy

Since the pituitary gland is a small midline tumor, the goal of treatment is to deliver a homogeneous dose to the preoperative adenoma and spare normal brain tissue. This is best done through multiple fields (two laterals and a vertex field), or arcs.

The target volume for the field should be enclosed within the 95% isodose line. For arc therapy, the patient is supine with the chin tucked so that when the gantry rotates, the beam does not traverse the superior orbit. This position can be achieved by elevating the patient's head with a head holder, or by placing the patient on a slant board. The field is generally centered on the sella, measuring 5x5 cm to 6x6 cm in size. Wedges are often used to deliver a homogeneous dose distribution.

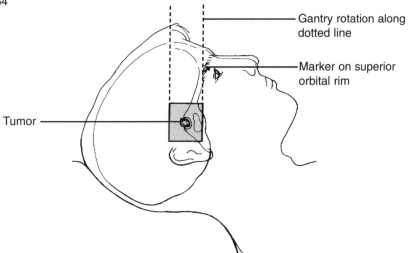

Gantry rotation along dotted line

Marker on superior orbital rim

Tumor

Fig. 2.6 Treatment Field for Tumor of the Pituitary

Dose

The dose delivered is generally 45-50 Gy at 1.8-2.0 Gy per fraction, and larger masses may require a boost to 54 Gy.

Chapter 3

Breast Cancer

Breast cancer is the most common malignancy in women in the United States. One of every nine females will have cancer of the breast during their life. There is an increased risk of breast cancer in women with a family history of this cancer and in women who are nulliparous. Early stage breast cancer can be successfully treated with conservative surgery followed by radiation treatments. Conservative surgery followed by radiation provides the same curability as mastectomy but without the psychological and physical loss of the breast. Mastectomy should be reserved for patients with extensive carcinoma (unable to be resected with clear margins and an acceptable cosmetic outcome), or patients who prefer this alternative.

Breast cancer arises from the epithelium of the ducts. The most common histology is infiltrating ductal, which accounts for 65-80% of all invasive breast cancers.

Anatomy

The adult breast extends vertically from the second to the sixth costal cartilage and horizontally from the edge of the sternum to the anterior axillary line. Breast tissue extends into the axilla as the axillary tail of Spence. The deep surface of the breast lies on the pectoralis major and serratus muscles.

Routes of Spread

The breast contains lymphatics which drain through three major pathways: the axillary, the internal mammary, and the transpectoral. Breast cancer also spreads by direct extension or through the dermal lymphatics in all directions.

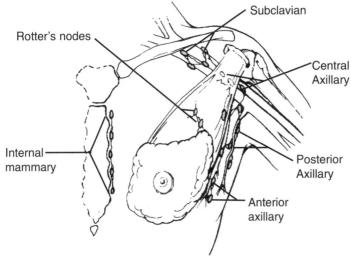

Figure 3.1 Lymph Nodes of the Breast

The internal mammary lymph nodes are located along the internal mammary arteries on both sides of the sternum approximately 3 cm lateral to the midline. They can be found at a depth of approximately 2.5-3 cm below the skin surface, in the intercostal spaces. The greatest concentration of internal mammary nodes is in the upper three interspaces. Involvement of the internal mammary nodes increases with central or medial tumors and proven axillary nodal metastases.

The transpectoral pathway passes through the pectoralis major muscle and drains into the supraclavicular lymph nodes. The supraclavicular lymph nodes are generally located superior to the clavicle and lateral to the sternocleidomastoid muscle (at <3 cm below the surface).

The major route of nodal drainage is through the axillary pathway. The axillary nodes are located near the patient's midline, at a depth of approximately 6-8 cm. The axillary lymph nodes are divided into three levels.

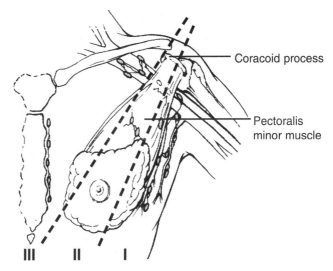

Fig. 3.2 Levels of the Axillary Lymph Nodes

Level I - nodes under the lower portion and lateral to the pectoralis minor muscle
Level II - directly under the pectoralis minor muscle
Level III -nodes superior to the pectoralis minor muscle

(Note: Level I-III nodes lie medial to the humeral head and do not extend laterally beyond the coracoid process. The nodes become more anterior as they extend superiomedially, i.e. levels I to II to III.)

Technical Aspects of Radiation Therapy
Conservative surgery and radiation therapy :

After wide resection with 1-2 cm margin of normal appearing breast tissue and an axillary dissection, the entire breast must be irradiated using tangential fields. A small margin of lung is included in the tangential fields so that the entire breast and chest wall are irradiated.

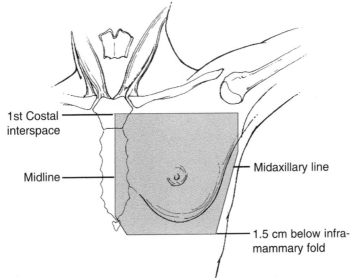

Fig. 3.3 Tangential Irradiation Field

The breast tangential portals are set up with the following borders:

Medial - midline
Lateral - mid-axillary line (2 cm beyond all breast tissue)
Superior - first costal interspace (or as superior as possible, may be limited by the ipsilateral arm)
Inferior - 1.5 cm below inframammary fold

Generally, patients are placed on a slant board to compensate for the slope of the sternum and chest wall. In some cases, the slant board can also prevent the breast from falling superiorly toward the supraclavicular area.

A boost to the surgical bed is commonly recommended

because microscopic tumor burden is greatest near the gross tumor mass. The boost may be given with an interstitial implant or electrons. When using electrons the 80% isodose line should be on the chest wall, or below the deepest part of the tylectomy cavity. Be aware that the lumpectomy site does not always lie directly under the surgical incision.

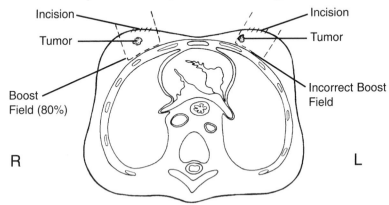

Figure 3.4 Comparison of Breast Boosts

A supraclavicular field is generally treated in patients with four or more positive axillary nodes or extracapsular extension.

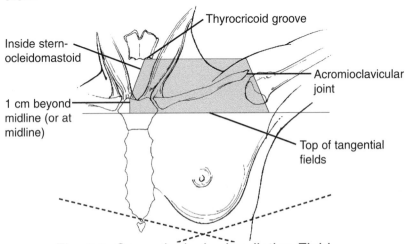

Fig. 3.5 Supraclavicular Irradiation Field

The supraclavicular field is set up with the following borders:

Medial - Vertical line 1 cm across the midline (or at midline) extending from the first costal interspace to the thyro- cricoid groove, medial to the sternocleidomastoid muscle to include the lower lymph nodes of the cervical chain. (These nodes lie under the sternocleidomastoid muscle and extend down to the insertion of the sternocleidomastoid muscle at the head of the clavicle).

Superior - Extends laterally across the neck and trapezius to the acromial process (make sure entire supraclavicular fossa is included visually).

Lateral - From the acromioclavicular joint, bisecting the humeral head, to exclude as much of the shoulder as possible. A custom cut block may be used to block the entire humeral head. (Remember: the axillary nodes lie medial to the humeral head and the coracoid process).

Inferior - At the first costal interspace, abutting the tangential breast field

The supraclavicular portal may be angled 10-15° to prevent exposure of the spinal cord and esophagus. The lower portion of the field is blocked with a matching half-beam block to eliminate overlap with the tangential field. When treating the tangential field, the table can be angled to match the superior border of the tangential field with the inferior border of the supraclavicular field to further prevent overlap. Depending on nodal status, a posterior axillary boost (PAB), may be considered (see indications for a PAB in the Postoperative Radiation Therapy section).

Dose

The breast tangents should be treated to 46.8-50.4 Gy (at 1.8-2.0 Gy per fraction), preferably using 4-6 mV photons. Wedges are often used to achieve dose homogeneity. Bolus is not recommended to the intact breast because the skin is not at risk for recurrence. The tumor bed is usually boosted to a dose of 60 Gy.

The supraclavicular field is treated anteriorly to 46.8 Gy at 1.8 Gy per fraction at a depth of 3 cm.

Postoperative Radiation Therapy

Postoperative radiation adjuvant therapy after a modified radical mastectomy, is used to eradicate microscopic foci and increase local control in patients who are at an increased risk for local recurrence. The chest wall may be treated through tangential fields or single or multiple electron fields. If the surgical incision or drain sites extend outside of the treatment field, these areas can be treated with electrons. In general, the guidelines for chest wall irradiation are similar to treating the intact breast. For patients in whom the internal mammary nodes are not irradiated, the field borders are identical to Figure 3.5.

Treatment of the internal mammary nodes is controversial. Local recurrence in this area is low. Therefore, when treating only to prevent local recurrence, the internal mammary nodes do not need to be included. When treating a patient comprehensively and trying to affect survival, the internal mammary nodes are generally treated. The internal mammary nodes should not be included in the tangential fields on a routine basis because of the increased morbidity associated with including additional heart and lung in the treatment portal. Furthermore, by placing the medial border of the tangential field 3 cm across the midline in an effort to include the internal mammary nodes, there is an increased potential of irradiating the opposite breast, as well as an increased inhomogeneity of the beam. It is also uncertain whether the internal mammary nodes are adequately included when using this tangential method. In cases where the treatment of internal mammary nodes is indicated, a separate internal mammary node portal should be designed rather than exposing more heart and lung in the tangential field.

Various techniques have been used for irradiation of the internal mammary nodes concurrently with the chest wall. A commonly used method is described as follows:

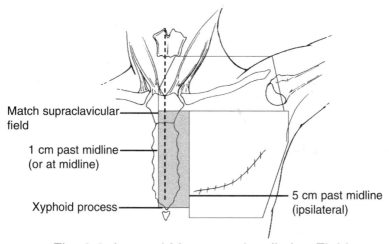

Match supraclavicular field

1 cm past midline (or at midline)

Xyphoid process

5 cm past midline (ipsilateral)

Fig. 3.6 Internal Mammary Irradiation Field

The borders of the internal mammary field are:
Superior - to match the supraclavicular field
Inferior - the xiphoid process
Medial - 1 cm past midline on the contralateral side (or to

midline)

Lateral - 5 cm past midline on the the ipsilateral side, to include the internal mammary nodes

The tangential fields are matched to the lateral internal mammary port.

To prevent excess irradiation to the mediastinum, a mixed beam portal can be used to treat the internal mammary nodes. An electron energy should be selected to deliver 90% of the dose to 4 cm (usually 12-15 MeV). Remember: the internal mammary nodes are located at approximately 3 cm depth. The electron beam can be angled 5 degrees less than the medial tangential beam to decrease the cold spot between the internal mammary and tangential portals.

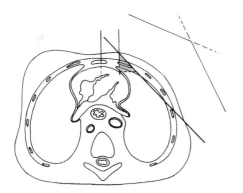

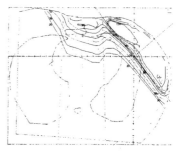

Fig. 3.7a Shaded area represents cold spot with anterior internal mammary node field.

Fig. 3.7b 5:1 15mev electrons: 6mv photons. Electrons angled 5° less than medial tangential field. Note: No cold spot. Medial border is actually 2 cm contralateral to midline when angling the electron field.

The supraclavicular field should be set up as described in the conservative surgery and radiation therapy section.

64

A posterior axillary portal can be used for patients with four or more positive axillary nodes, greater than 2.5 cm nodes, fixed nodes, extranodal extension, or an inadequately dissected axilla. This field is treated posteriorly to raise the dose in the midline and posterior axillary nodes that would have been underdosed because of the fall off of dose in the supraclavicular/axillary field.

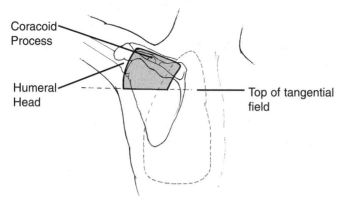

Fig. 3.8 Posterior Axillary Boost

The borders of the PAB are as follows:
Superior - bisect the clavicle and bisect the humeral head
Inferior - the field matches the superior border of the tangential field
Medial - to include the axillary nodes that lie close to the chest wall (a small margin of the lung is necessary). Remember: the level III nodes lie medial to the coracoid process and the level II nodes are medial to the humeral head.
Lateral - the latissimus dorsi muscle

Dose

The chest wall is treated to 50.4 Gy (at 1.8-2.0 Gy per fraction). Patients with close margins, recurrent disease, or advanced primary tumors should be boosted with electrons to the surgical scar to 60 Gy. A 0.5-1 cm bolus may be used every other day (or every third day) to increase the surface dose to the skin. Use of bolus is especially important in patients with recurrent or inflammatory breast cancer.

The supraclavicular field is treated anteriorly to 46.8 Gy at 1.8 Gy per fraction, to a depth of 3 cm. The posterior axillary field can be added to bring the midline axillary dose to the prescribed 46.8 Gy.

Chapter 4

Hodgkin's Disease

Hodgkin's disease was first identified in 1832 by the pathologist, Thomas Hodgkin. There is a bi-modal age specific incidence of Hodgkin's disease with one peak occurring between 15-24 years and the second after the age 50. The diagnosis of Hodgkin's disease is dependent upon the identification of the Reed-Sternberg cell which is a large, irregular cell with a multi-lobed nucleus. The most common presenting symptom of patients diagnosed with Hodgkin's disease is a painless enlargement of a lymph node. Other symptoms which may be present and adversely affect the prognosis include fever, night sweats and weight loss.

Anatomy

At the time of diagnosis, Hodgkin's disease is usually found to be localized, or involve contiguous nodal groups. At presentation, greater than 75% of patients will have cervical or supraclavicular lymphadenopathy and 60% will have involvement of the mediastinum. The Ann Arbor staging system for Hodgkin's disease is based upon the lymph node areas involved and the presence or absence of systemic symptoms which include fever, night sweats and weight loss.

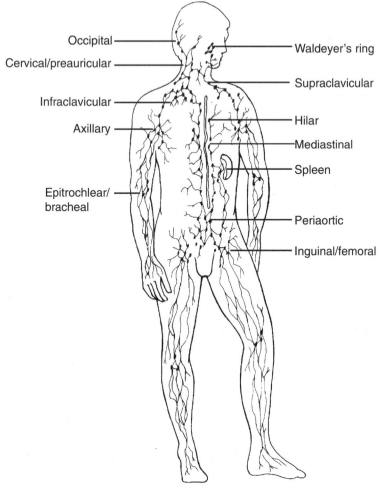

Fig. 4.1 Lymph Node Regions in Hodgkin's Disease

Treatment of Hodgkin's Disease

Hodgkin's disease is extremely radiosensitive. The advent of the use of high energy x-rays in the treatment of Hodgkin's disease has resulted in a dramatic increase in the curability of this disease. It is now considered to be among the most curable of all cancers.

Surgery is primarily used to obtain tissue for diagnosis. A staging laparotomy with a splenectomy will be performed only if the findings of the laparotomy will influence the decision regarding the best treatment method for the patient. In female patients, an oophoropexy is performed at the time of laparotomy. This is a surgical technique of moving the ovaries to the patient's midline, posterior to the uterus, in order to shield the ovaries from radiation and maintain reproductive function.

Radiation therapy is the treatment of choice in early stage Hodgkin's disease. Radiation is used to treat all of the involved, and the potentially involved lymph nodes, in order to sterilize all sites of disease. The contiguous pattern of spread in Hodgkin's disease must be considered when determining the areas to be encompassed within radiation therapy treatment portals. Chemotherapy alone, or in combination with radiation, is used for more advanced disease.

Technical Aspects of Radiation Therapy

In order to optimally treat Hodgkin's disease, the radiation oncology department must be equipped with a high energy linear accelerator, a simulator, a block cutter for customized blocks, and a modern treatment planning computer.

AP/PA Mantle Field
Treatment of the lymph node areas above the diaphragm is termed the mantle field. The nodal groups included in the mantle field are the cervical, submandibular, axillary, supra-clavicular, infraclavicular, mediastinal, and hilar lymph nodes.

Patients are treated supine with their arms above their head, or on their hips, and their chin extended. No head cushion is used. The central axis of the beam is generally located at the suprasternal notch.

A typical AP and PA mantle port is shown below. In addition to the lung, humeral head and occipital blocks, anterior larynx and posterior spinal cord blocks are usually added. Modifications in portal size and field blocking can be made based on the stage and extent of the disease.

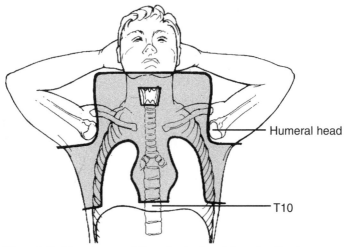

Fig. 4.2 Borders of the Anterior Mantle Port

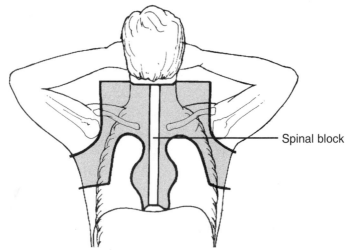

Fig. 4.3 Borders of the Posterior Mantle Port

Borders of the Mantle Field are:

Superior - lower mandible and the mastoid tips (the chin must be extended so that the high cervical and submandibular nodes are included in the port, without treating the mouth

Inferior - T9-T10 interspace or insertion of the diaphragm

Lateral - fall-off, to include the axillary nodes

Note: More recently, linear accelerators with the extended range treatment couches and larger field sizes have allowed patients to be treated supine with the gantry rotating under for the parallel opposed field rather than "flipping" the patient over for the posterior field. When the patient is "flipped" to the prone position, the chin must remain extended. It is also difficult, but necessary, to match the central ray and the caudal margin of the posterior port to that of the anterior port.

The extent of treatment of the subdiaphragmatic nodes is individualized based upon the stage of disease and findings at laparotomy.

AP/PA Inverted Y Ports

An inverted Y port consists of the following nodals groups: the retroperitoneal or periaortic nodes, the pelvic nodes, the spleen, or splenic hilar nodes, and the femoral nodes. When treatment of all of these areas is indicated, this large port is usually divided into abdominal and pelvic ports for sequential treatment. Separating the large treatment volume is usually better tolerated by the patient.

Subtotal nodal irradiation consists of irradiation of the mantle field and the abdominal (or periaortic) portion of the inverted Y. Addition of the pelvic ports to the mantle and the abdominal ports is termed total nodal irradiation.

If a mantle field was treated, the patient should be placed in the same treatment position. Precise calculation and film verification of a gap must be recorded to eliminate any potential overlap of treatment fields on the spinal cord. In addition to the calculations and film verification, a small spinal cord block may be placed superiorly at the junction of the mantle and subdiaphragmatic ports. Renal contrast and opacified lymph nodes from the lymphangiogram are helpful in defining the lateral treatment borders, especially when the entire spleen must be treated. When treating the spleen, or splenic pedicle, the left kidney should be protected as much as possible. In certain cases, treatment of the liver is indicated. This can be achieved with a partial liver transmission block.

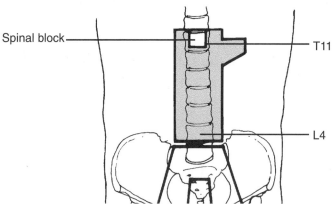

Fig. 4.4 Borders of the Abdominal (Periaortic) Port

Borders of the Abdominal (Periaortic) portion of the Inverted Y:

Superior - Approximately mid T-10, with an appropriate gap from the mantle field

Inferior - L4-L5

Lateral - usually 9-10 cm wide, (blocks may be cut to encompass the spleen or splenic pedicle)

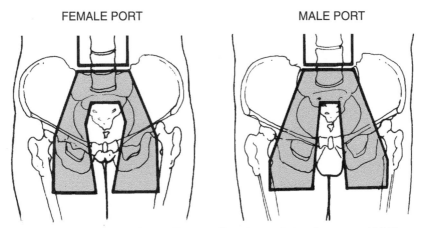

FEMALE PORT   MALE PORT

Fig. 4.5 Borders of the Pelvic Portion of the Inverted Y Port

Borders of the Pelvic Portion of the Inverted Y are:
Superior - L-5 with an appropriate gap from the abdominal
port
Inferior - 2 cm below the ischial tuberosity to include the
femoral nodes
Lateral - 2 cm beyond the pelvic inlet (exclude as much of
the pelvis as possible while leaving an adequate
margin around the lymphatics)

Treatment of the pelvis requires special consideration of
fertility and gonadal shielding. Oophoropexy in the female
as previously described moves the ovaries away from their
normal position overlying the iliac nodes to a position in
the midline which can be effectively blocked. In the male, a
gonadal shield will significantly decrease the dose to the
testes.

Dose

Many studies and discussions have attempted to document
the appropriate doses for Hodgkin's disease; however, con-

troversy remains concerning the optimum total doses. Most radiation oncologists agree that total doses of 36-44 Gy at fractions of 1.8-2.0 Gy will eradicate gross disease, whereas, a minimum of 30-36 Gy is recommended for microscopic disease.

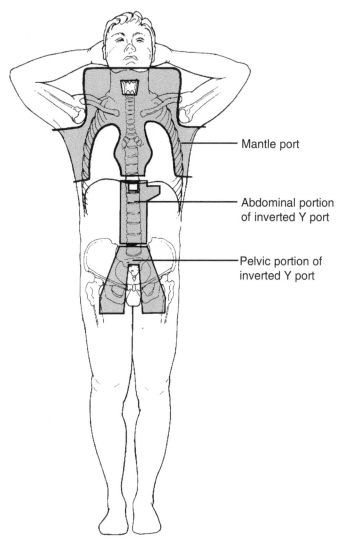

Mantle port

Abdominal portion of inverted Y port

Pelvic portion of inverted Y port

Chapter 5

Lung Cancer

Lung cancer is the leading cause of cancer related deaths in both males and females. Approximately 10% of patients with lung cancer will survive five years.

Anatomy

The right lung is divided into three lobes and the left lung is divided into two lobes. The trachea branches into the right and left mainstem bronchi at the level of the fifth thoracic vertebra. The lungs are separated in the midline by the mediastinum which is composed of the heart, thymus, trachea, great vessels, esophagus, and lymph nodes. The medi-

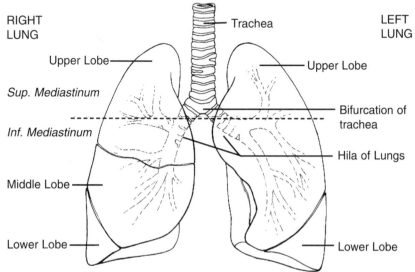

Fig. 5.1 Anatomy of the Lungs

astinum can be divided into superior and inferior compart-
ments (above and below the level of the bifurcation of the
trachea). The hila of the lungs contain blood vessels,
bronchi and lymphatics.

Routes of Spread

The primary routes of tumor spread include the lymphatics,
blood vessels and direct extension (intrathoracic). Involvement of the lymphatics tends to occur early and follows the
divisions of the bronchial tree. The intrapulmonary nodes
along the segmental bronchi are initially involved, followed
by spread to the hilar nodes. The lymphatic channels then
drain to the mediastinal nodes and ultimately to the supraclavicular nodes.

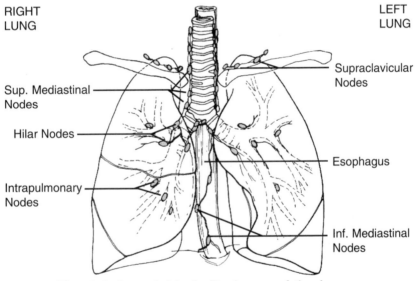

Fig. 5.2 Lymph Node Drainage of the Lungs

Treatment Options

For general treatment purposes, cancer of the lung can be

divided into two categories based on its histopathology: non-small cell and small cell carcinoma. In early stages of non-small cell cancer, when the tumor is localized, surgery is the treatment of choice. If the non-small tumor is inoperable (due to its size, location, or regional lymph node involvement) and has not metastisized, high dose radiation should be offered for optimal control. There is a direct correlation between the dose of radiation and local control in lung cancer.

Small cell cancer of the lung spreads rapidly, and has a high probability of metastasis at the time of diagnosis. Because of its rapid dissemination, multiagent chemotherapy and radiation therapy offer the best chance for a complete response. Many new protocols have shown a definite advantage to irradiating the chest simultaneously with the administration of multiagent chemotherapy.

Technical Aspects of Radiation Therapy

The treatment portal is designed based on the size of the primary tumor, location, and the lymphatic drainage. Overall, ipsilateral hilar nodes are involved in 50-60%, mediastinal nodes in 40-50%, and supraclavicular nodes in 5-30% of patients. The risk of supraclavicular nodal involvement increases when there is disease involving the superior mediastinal nodes, or upper lobes of the lungs. Treatment portals are usually designed with a 2 cm margin around both the primary tumor and the nodal areas which are involved, or at risk. Irregular fields with cut blocks are almost always used. Based on tumor location and potential lymphatic involvement, treatment portals can be designed as follows:

1) Tumor involvement of the upper lobes

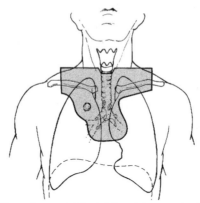

Fig. 5.3 Treatment Field for Upper Lobe Tumor

Treatment portal includes the primary tumor, both hilar areas, superior mediastinum, and both supraclavicular areas.

2) Tumor involvement of middle lobes with mediastinal nodes:

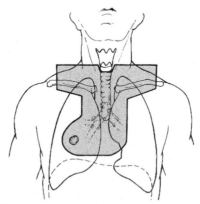

Fig. 5.4 Treatment Field for Middle Lobe Tumor

Treatment portal includes the primary tumor, both hilar areas, superior mediastinum, and both supraclavicular areas.

3) Tumor involvement of middle lobes without mediastinal nodes:

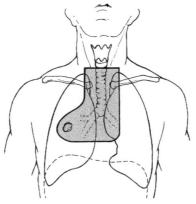

Fig. 5.5 Treatment Field for Middle Lobe Tumor (no nodes)

Treatment portal includes the primary tumor, both hilar areas, and superior mediastinum.

4) Tumor involvement of the lower lobes without mediastinal nodes:

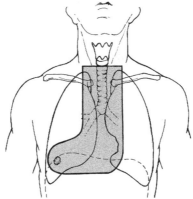

Fig. 5.6 Treatment Field for Lower Lobe Tumor

Treatment portal includes the primary tumor and entire mediastinum.

5) If there is evidence of mediastinal adenopathy, generally both supraclavicular areas are included in the treatment portal.

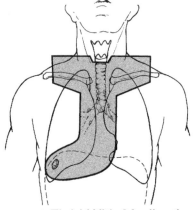

Fig. 5.7 Treatment Field With Mediastinal Adenopathy

Dose

Initially, treatment portals are treated AP-PA to doses of 40-45 Gy. Oblique portals are often used to boost the tumor, to avoid exceeding the tolerance to sensitive structures such as lung, spinal cord and heart. Total doses of 65-70 Gy are employed to the primary tumor and areas of gross disease.

Chapter 6

Gastrointestinal Cancer

THE ESOPHAGUS

Cancer of the esophagus accounts for only 1% of all cancers in the United States. The overall prognosis for cancer of the esophagus remains very poor with cure rates less than 10%. The incidence of esophageal cancer is higher in males than females and the major histologic type is squamous cell carcinoma.

Anatomy

The esophagus is a hollow tube of squamous epithelium, measuring 20-25 cm. A muscular wall surrounds the inner mucosa layer. The esophagus lacks an outer coating, or serosal layer.

The esophagus is usually divided into :
1) the cervical esophagus - extending from the cricoid cartilage to the thoracic inlet (level of T1)
2) upper thoracic - thoracic inlet to the bifurcation of the trachea
3) middle thoracic - proximal half of the esophagus between the bifurcation of the trachea and the gastroesophageal junction.
4) lower thoracic - distal half of the esophagus between the bifurcation of the trachea and the gastroesophageal junction.

Anatomical Landmarks and Divisions of the Esophagus

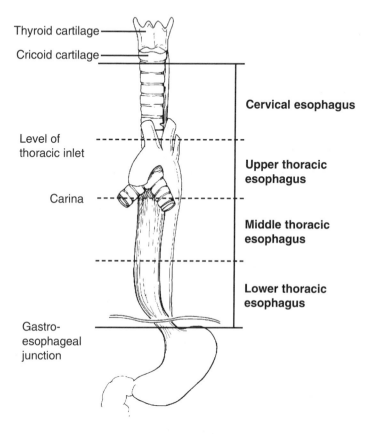

Thyroid cartilage

Cricoid cartilage

Cervical esophagus

Level of
thoracic inlet

**Upper thoracic
esophagus**

Carina

**Middle thoracic
esophagus**

**Lower thoracic
esophagus**

Gastro-
esophageal
junction

Fig. 6.1   Anatomical Divisions of the Esophagus

Routes of Spread

The esophagus contains a rich lymphatic network that
interconnects throughout the length of the esophagus and
generally spreads in a longitudinal course. Cancer cells may
spread to any portion of the esophagus as well as to lymph
nodes in the neck, thorax and upper abdomen. Tumors of

the upper esophagus spread most commonly to the internal jugular, cervical, or supraclavicular lymph nodes. Middle esophageal tumors disseminate primarily to the supraclavicular, paratracheal and mediastinal nodes. Lower esophageal tumors generally involve the lower mediastinal, gastric, and celiac axis nodes.

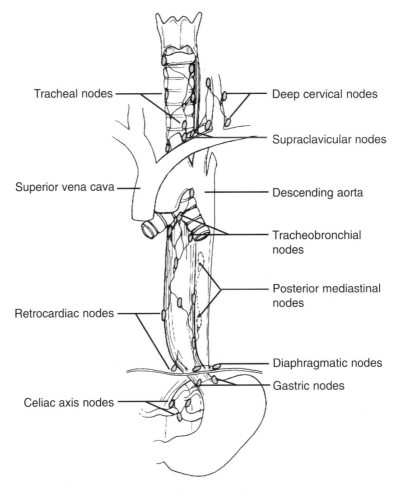

Fig. 6.2   Lymph Drainage of the Esophagus

Without a serosal layer, tumors of the esophagus may spread very easily to contiguous structures in the mediastinum. Also distant metastases via hematogenous spread is common and can occur early. Hematogenous spread to the liver, lungs and bones may be found in 40% of the patients at the time of diagnosis.

Technical Aspects of Radiation Therapy

Historically, if tumors were found localized in the esophagus with no evidence of metastases, surgery was the primary treatment. However, because of the high incidence of both local and distant spread, the results with surgery alone have been poor. External beam radiation therapy can be used alone in a curative manner for localized tumors or as a palliative measure to help relieve symptoms or obstruction. Recently, studies have combined chemotherapy and radiation therapy or chemotherapy, radiation therapy and surgery in an attempt to improve local control and cure rates. Patients who are found to have a complete response to chemotherapy and radiation have shown improved two and three year survival rates.

When considering the patient with cancer of the esophagus for treatment with radiation either palliatively or radically, an adequate treatment volume must be defined with at least a 5-6 cm margin above and below the tumor. Anterior-posterior and lateral simulation films with barium will help to define the tumor volume. Because of the close proximity of critical structures such as the heart, lungs and spinal cord, careful treatment planning and patient positioning must be observed. Also, consideration must be given to the natural contour of the neck and thorax when planning a long treatment portal. If possible, CT treatment planning should be performed and the tumor volume outlined, so that different field arrangements can be tried. Treatment techniques for the cervical esophagus include lateral parallel opposed or oblique portals. Another technique utilizes a four field box with wax bolus above the shoulders to act as a compensator. Lateral portals may then be used as a boost to the primary.

For tumors of the thoracic esophagus, treatment techniques include: AP-PA fields, oblique portals, arc rotations or a combination of the above. Most institutions initially treat an AP-PA portal using high energy photons to doses of 30-40 Gy. In order to spare the spinal cord two posterior obliques may then be used as a boost.

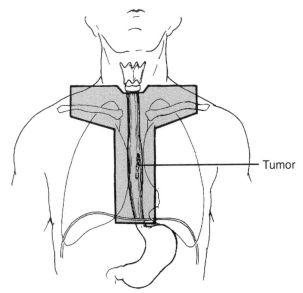

Fig. 6.3 Esophageal Treatment Field

Cervical Esophagus Port:
Superior - laryngopharynx or 5 cm above the
                tumor
Inferior - carina or 5-6 cm below the tumor volume

The anterior cervical, superior mediastinal and supraclavicular nodes are usually included in the treatment volume.

Thoracic Esophageal Port:
Superior - 5-6 cm above the tumor volume
Inferior - 5-6 cm below the tumor volume
The treatment port usually includes the entire thoracic esophagus.

For lower thoracic esophageal tumors, the treatment port is extended to include the celiac axis nodes.

Doses

Palliative treatment for cancer of the esophagus consists of doses that range from 30 Gy over two weeks to 50 Gy over 5 weeks. Preoperative doses of 30 Gy over three weeks to 45 Gy over 5 weeks have been used in combination with chemotherapy. For patients where surgery is not planned, boosts to 60-65 Gy are usually recommended. In addition to external beam, both low dose rate intracavitary therapy (LDR) and high dose rate intracavitary therapy (HDR) have been used for both palliative and radical treatment. Many treatment plans utilize HDR intraluminal brachytherapy with Ir-192 as a boost following external beam.

STOMACH CANCER

Although the incidence of stomach cancer is high in Japan, the incidence and mortality in the United States has declined over the past 50 years. Dietary factors such as smoked foods have been implicated as a risk factor in gastric cancer. Pathologically, most gastric cancers are ulcerative adenocarcinomas. Patients diagnosed with gastric cancer generally complain of weight loss, decreased appetite, abdominal pain and nausea and vomiting.

Anatomy

The stomach is made up of a muscular wall with a mucosal lining which contains a variety of different types of cells exhibiting different radiosensitivity. The stomach begins at the gastroesophageal junction and ends at the pylorus, which joins the duodenum. The stomach is surrounded by a number of vital structures including the liver, transverse colon, left kidney, pancreas, left adrenal, spleen, and various segments of the small bowel.

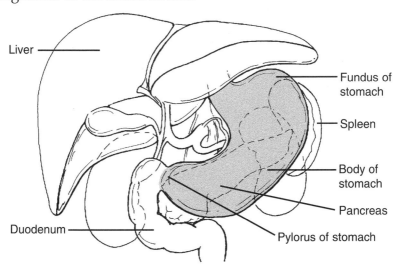

Fig. 6.4 Anatomy of the Stomach

Routes of Spread

There are four primary routes of spread for gastric carcinoma. These tumors can spread by direct extension to adjacent organs and viscera. Widespread dissemination occurs by way of the lymphatics, hematogenous spread, or by spillage into the peritoneal cavity.

The stomach contains a rich lymphatic network that connects and flows through three major pathways. The lymphatics can drain through the left gastric trunk, the splenic collecting trunk, or the hepatic collecting trunk. Splenic nodal groups that are at risk for metastatic spread include the gastric, gastropancreatic, celiac axis, and the adjacent periaortic nodes.

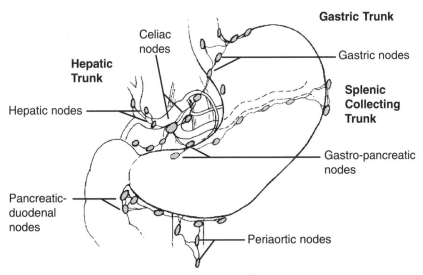

Fig. 6.5   Lymph Drainage of the Stomach

Treatment

In cases where the tumor is limited to the stomach, the treatment of choice is a radical subtotal gastrectomy with the removal of adjacent nodal tissue. Gastric cancer has a high propensity for locoregional failure. The tumor bed and regional lymph nodes are at greatest risk for recurrence. Distant metastases are also common with advanced disease, and often involve the liver and lungs.

Because of the high rate of locoregional failure following surgery, especially in cases where the tumor extends through the wall of the stomach or positive lymph nodes are found, radiation therapy has been used postoperatively. Post-op radiation, usually combined with chemotherapy, has proven to be beneficial in local control of the primary tumor. In unresectable cases, radiation has been successful in the palliation of gastric cancer symptoms.

Technical Aspects of Radiation Therapy

Radiation portals must be designed with careful consideration of the surrounding dose limiting structures. The radiation portal should include the tumor bed and the major surrounding lymphatic groups. AP/PA portals, using beam energies of 6 mV or greater, are typically employed.

Treatment Borders for Cancer of the Stomach:
Superior - 3-4 cm margin around the tumor or tumor bed
Inferior - bottom of L3
Lateral - 3-4 cm margin around the tumor or tumor bed and primary nodal groups with special contouring of the port to exclude three-fourths of one kidney

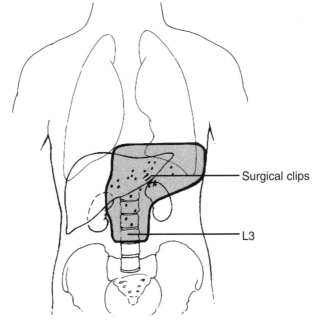

Fig. 6.6 Postoperative Portal for Cancer of the Stomach

Dose

Generally, doses of 40-45 Gy at 1.8 Gy per fraction are given to a large AP/PA portal in combination with concurrent chemotherapy (5FU). This treatment portal and the doses can be used either for adjuvant postoperative treatment, or treatment for palliation of symptoms. Small boost ports may be treated to 50-55 Gy for areas of residual or gross disease.

CANCER OF THE PANCREAS

The incidence and the mortality rate of pancreatic cancer continues to increase and parallel one another very closely. Several factors associated with an increased risk of pancreatic cancer include cigarette smoking, alcohol consumption, and chronic pancreatitis. The majority of pancreatic cancers are ductal adenocarcinomas and occur in the head of the pancreas.

Anatomy

The pancreas is found in the posterior peritoneum. It is composed of three parts designated the head, the body and the tail. The head of the pancreas is overlapped by the duodenum at approximately the level of the first two lumbar vertebrae. The tail of the pancreas extends to the splenic hilum.

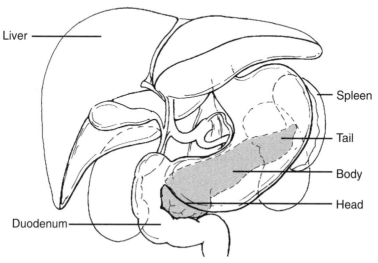

Fig. 6.7 The Pancreas

Routes of Spread

Because of the rich lymphatic network of the pancreas, several nodal groups are at risk for metastatic involvement. Those at greatest risk include the superior and inferior pancreaticoduodenal, the porta hepatis, the suprapancreatic and the adjacent periaortic nodes. Pancreatic tumors tend to spread by direct extension to adjacent vital structures including the bile duct system, the stomach and the duodenum. Hematogenous metastases are common and usually involve the liver, lungs or pleura.

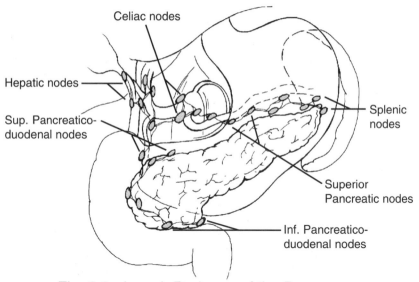

Fig. 6.8   Lymph Drainage of the Pancreas

Treatment

The treatment of choice for localized pancreatic cancer is surgical resection. Unfortunately, only about 10-25% of patients are candidates for surgery with curative intent. To date, 5 year survival rates remain very poor (5-10%).

For patients able to undergo surgery, there is evidence to support the use of postoperative radiation therapy in combination with 5FU chemotherapy. By irradiating the tumor bed and surrounding nodal areas, the risk of local recurrence can be decreased and survival possibly improved.

For patients with unresectable pancreatic cancers, palliation can be achieved using combined external beam radiation and chemotherapy.

Technical Aspects of Radiation Therapy

Due to the proximity of the pancreas to critical dose limiting structures (such as the liver, small bowel, stomach, kidney and spinal cord), a multi-field technique, using high energy photons, should be employed.

The treatment volume can be determined by post-surgical clips, MRI or CT scans (with the patient in the treatment position), endoscopic studies, or ultrasonography. The patient should be treated supine. A 2-3 cm margin should be planned around the tumor bed, or primary tumor, to include adjacent pancreatic tissue and major nodal groups. Renal contrast is necessary for precise localization of the kidneys, and barium can be used to delineate the duodenum. The portal should be planned to respect the tolerance of all surrounding radiosensitive structures, particularly the liver and the kidneys.

Either a three field (AP, right and left lateral) or a four field (AP/PA, right and left lateral) technique can be used. The treatment technique will vary depending on the following factors: the location, size and extent of the tumor or tumor bed, and the location of critical structures in relation to the treatment volume. The dose to the kidney and spine can be reduced by treating through an anterior and two lateral fields only. Appropriate field weighting is necessary to deliver an adequate dose to the tumor volume, while respecting the dose to critical surrounding structures.

Treatment Borders for Tumors Involving the Head of the Pancreas:

The treatment portal for tumors located in the head of the pancreas should include the following nodal groups: the pancreaticoduodenal, the porta hepatis, the celiac, and the suprapancreatic.

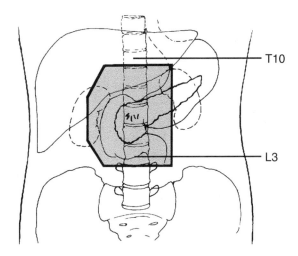

Fig. 6.9 AP Treatment Port for Tumor in Head of Pancreas

Borders for the AP or AP/PA port(s):
Superior - T11-T12 or a 2-3 cm margin around the tumor or the tumor bed
Inferior - bottom of L3
Lateral - 2-3 cm margin around the tumor or the tumor bed with exclusion of at least three-fourths of the left kidney. You may need to include at least 50% of the right kidney as well as the duodenum.

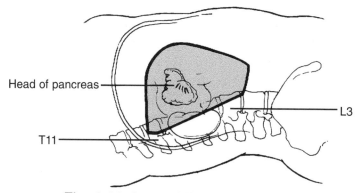

Fig. 6.10 Lateral Pancreatic Treatment Port

Borders for the Lateral Ports:
Anterior - 1-2 cm beyond the tumor or tumor bed
Posterior - split the vertebral bodies

Treatment Borders for Pancreatic Body or Tail Tumors

Treatment portals for tumors arising in the body or the tail of the pancreas should include the pancreaticoduodenal nodes, the porta hepatis nodes, and the splenic hilar nodes.

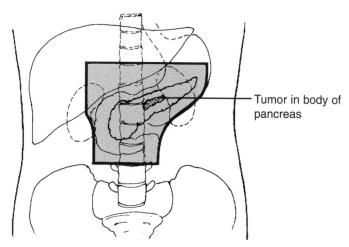

Fig. 6.11 Treatment Port for Tumor in Body/Tail of Pancreas

Borders for the AP or AP/PA port(s):
Superior - top of T11
Inferior - bottom of L3
Lateral - exclude at least two-thirds of the right kidney. It is not necessary to include the entire duodenal loop. The port is extended to the left to obtain a 3 cm margin around the tumor and to include the splenic hilum.

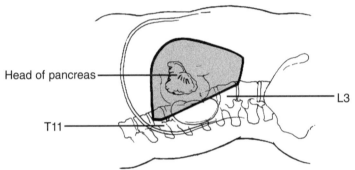

Fig. 6.10 Lateral Pancreatic Treatment Port

Borders for the Lateral Ports:
Anterior - 1-2 cm beyond the tumor or tumor bed
Posterior - split the vertebral bodies

Dose

Doses of 45-50 Gy in 1.8 Gy per fraction in combination with 5FU chemotherapy have been used with acceptable tolerance. The contribution from the lateral treatment portal is limited to 18-20 Gy, secondary to the amount of liver and kidney volume in the treatment port.

Split course treatment has been used in palliative cases. Generally, a total of 60 Gy is delivered in 3 two week courses (20 Gy in two weeks, rest two weeks, then repeat). Field reduction is recommended after 45-50 Gy.

CARCINOMA OF THE RECTUM

In the United States, carcinoma of the rectum is the second most common cause of cancer related death. It occurs equally in men and women. The majority of patients are 50 years of age or older and they most commonly present with rectal bleeding. The majority of rectal cancers are adenocarcinomas which arise from the rectal mucosa.

Anatomy

The rectum is located between the sigmoid colon proximally and the anus distally. It is 13-15 cm in length. The rectum can be divided into three sections by the upper, middle and lower valves of Houston. The rectum and sigmoid colon join at approximately the level of S3. The rectum is closely associated with the sacral curve posteriorly. It is bounded by the vagina anteriorly in the female and by the trigone of the bladder, seminal vesicles, and prostate in the male. The

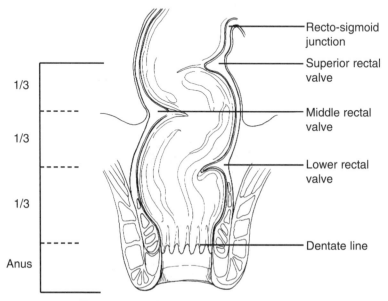

Fig. 6.13 Anatomy of the Rectum

rectum ends distally at the pectinate or dentate line, where the transition from rectal mucosa to squamous epithelium occurs.

Routes of Spread

Rectal cancer can spread by four pathways. Spread can occur by direct extension through the bowel wall to contiguous structures or organs. Widespread dissemination occurs by way of the lymphatics, hematogenous spread, or by transperitoneal implantation at the time of surgery.

Longitudinal tumor growth within the bowel wall generally occurs only for very short distances. Rectal tumors most often grow in an angular pattern, with extension into and through the layers of the bowel wall. Lymphatic drainage for the upper rectum follows the superior rectal vessels and terminates in the inferior mesenteric nodes. The middle and lower rectal lymphatics drain to the internal iliac and presacral nodes. If the lesion extends to the anal canal the

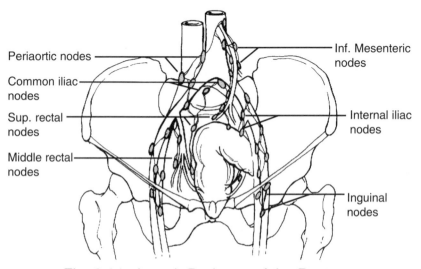

Fig. 6.14   Lymph Drainage of the Rectum

inguinal nodes may also be at risk. Hematogenous spread to the liver and lungs occurs most often with high grade tumors, and in those cases with lymphatic involvement. The liver is the most common site of metastatic spread.

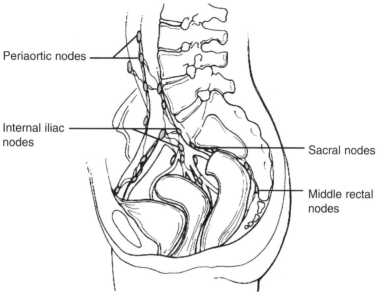

Fig. 6.15 Lymph Drainage of the Rectum (Lateral View)

Treatment

The treatment of choice for rectal cancer is surgical removal of the primary tumor and the primary nodal drainage. For tumors less than 6 cm from the anal verge, abdominoperineal resection with colostomy is required. In cases with rectal tumors greater than 6 cm from the anal verge, it is usually technically possible to perform a low anterior resection of the bowel with anastomosis. Local-regional failure is common in rectal cancer, especially for tumors extending through the bowel wall or involving regional lymphatics. For these reasons, radiation therapy and chemotherapy have been accepted as adjuvant treatment to improve the local control and survival of patients.

Radiation therapy has been used preoperatively, postoperatively, and both pre- and postoperatively (sandwich technique) in the treatment of rectal cancer.

Preoperative radiation therapy has the advantages of decreasing the viability of tumor cells that could spread at the time of surgery, improving the ability to resect large tumors, and decreasing the small bowel complications by radiating in a nonsurgical area.

Postoperative radiation has the advantage of better selection of patients for treatment based on the surgical pathologic findings.

Technical Aspects of Radiation Therapy

Whether preoperative or postoperative radiation therapy is used, the goal of treatment is to include the primary tumor or tumor bed with a 4-5 cm margin as well as the primary nodal drainage which generally includes the internal iliac and presacral nodes. The external iliac nodes are not generally included in the treatment port unless there is tumor involvement of other pelvic organs such as the vagina, bladder or uterus which may place these nodes at risk for metastases. In cases where postoperative radiation therapy is used following abdominoperineal resection (APR), the treatment portal must be extended to cover the perineum and surgical scar. Both four field and three field (posterior and two laterals) treatment ports have been used successfully.

Portal design depends on the location of the primary tumor, risk of adjacent nodal involvement, and presence of adjacent organ involvement. However, the following generalizations are commonly employed in treatment portal arrangement. The three field treatment technique is most commonly used and will be described here.

Patients are treated in the prone position so that the lateral ports can adequately encompass the posterior portion of the sacrum.

For patients receiving postoperative radiation, oral contrast may be given several hours prior to simulation in order to assess the amount of small bowel in the treatment portal. Both surgical and radiation techniques have been utilized to reduce the amount of small bowel in the treatment volume. These methods include pelvic reconstruction with reperitonealization, treating the patient prone with bladder distension, or a special small bowel displacement board used to allow the bowel to fall away from the pelvis.

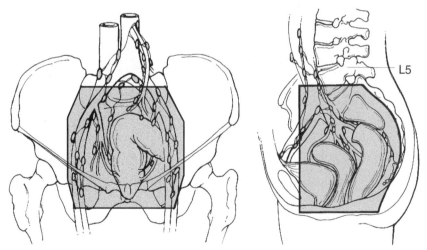

Fig. 6.16 PA and Lateral Treatment Ports for Rectal Cancer Following Low Anterior Resection

PA Field Borders:
Superior - bottom of L5
Inferior - at least 5 cm below the tumor (may need to include the anal margin for low rectal tumors)

Lateral - 1-2 cm beyond the pelvic inlet

Lateral Field Borders:
Posterior - posterior to the sacrum
Anterior - anterior to or mid-acetabulum (inclusion of the vagina is necessary in the female patient)

Following APR, it is important to include the perineum in the treatment portal in order to decrease the risk of a perineal recurrence secondary to tumor implantation at the time of surgery. The perineal scar is usually marked with a radiopaque marker at the time of simulation.

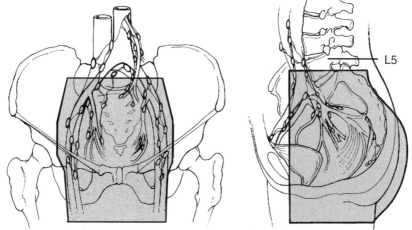

Fig. 6.17 PA and Lateral Treatment Ports following APR

PA Field Borders
Superior - bottom of L5
Inferior - 1-2 cm below the perineal scar
Lateral - 1-2 cm beyond the pelvic inlet
NOTE: when treating the posterior port the scar should be bolused.

Lateral Field Borders
Posterior - 1-2 cm beyond the perineal scar
Anterior - anterior to or mid-acetabulum

Doses

Doses of 45 Gy at 1.8 Gy per fraction are commonly used both preoperatively and postoperatively for carcinoma of the rectum. Field reduction and boost to 50 Gy may be considered for locally advanced tumors. Boost portals are best defined by preoperative barium studies and/or clip placement.

ANAL CANCER

Cancers of the anal region are uncommon in comparison to other bowel tumors and are predominantly squamous cell carcinomas. Anal carcinomas have been associated with condylomas or genital warts, anal intercourse in men, genital infections, and other causes of chronic irritation.

Anatomy

The anal canal measures approximately 3 cm in length and

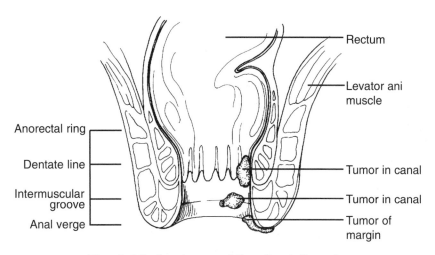

Fig. 6.18 Anatomy of the Anal Canal

extends from the anorectal ring superiorly to the anal verge inferiorly. The anal margin is defined as an area 5-6 cm in size surrounding the anal verge.

Routes of Spread

Anal cancers can spread by direct extension, lymphatics or the bloodstream. Hematogenous spread at the time of diagnosis is rare. Direct extension of anal cancers can involve the sphincter muscles, rectal wall, perianal skin, vaginal septum, prostate gland, sacrum and coccyx. Lymphatic spread from anal carcinomas occurs via three pathways. Tumors of the anal margin, anal verge and lower anal canal spread to the inguinal nodes. Carcinomas of the anal canal may also spread upward to the external and internal iliac nodes of the pelvis. Tumors of the upper anal canal and transition zone between the rectum and the anus may travel to the inferior mesenteric nodes. Hematogenous metastases may occur to the liver and the lungs.

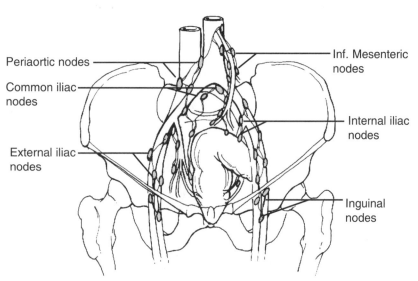

Fig. 6.19 Lymph Drainage of the Anus

Technical Aspects of Radiation Therapy

Historically, radical surgery, to include abdominoperineal resection, was the primary treatment for anal cancers. The use of combined radiation therapy and chemotherapy has resulted in a major treatment alternative in anal cancer and has improved survival, local control and sphincter preservation. Radical radiation therapy alone has also been used successfully especially with smaller tumors of the anus. Currently, most oncologists prefer treatment protocols using chemotherapy and radiation, reserving radical surgery for residual or recurrent disease. To date, the exact chemotherapy combination, as well as radiation dose schedule and portal design, has not been resolved. In spite of the variation in radiation portal design and dose schedules among institutions, the results of tumor control and survival are comparable.

For anal carcinomas, a combination of external beam therapy using megavoltage equipment with concurrent chemotherapy (5-FU and Mitomycin C) is used at our institution. Treatment portals are designed to include the primary tumor and regional nodes. Patients are simulated supine to allow visualization of the inguinal areas and a radiopaque marker is placed on the inferior most extension of the tumor or anal verge. For larger tumors, especially those greater than 5 cm, cone down boost ports to include the primary tumor are treated.

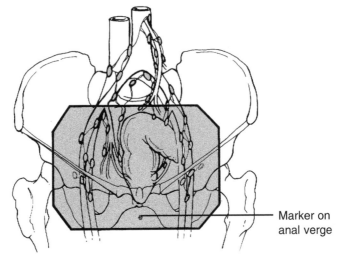

Marker on
anal verge

Fig. 6.20 Treatment Port for Cancer of the Anus

Borders of the treatment portal are as follows:
Superior - lower border of the sacroiliac joints
Inferior - 3 cm distal to the primary tumor
Lateral -   inclusion of the inguinal nodes

Doses

Generally, doses of 45 Gy at 1.8 Gy per fraction are given in combination with chemotherapy.

For larger anal carcinomas, boosts of 5-10 Gy may be given to treatment portals to include the primary tumor with a 2 cm margin.

For small tumors where radiation therapy alone may be considered, boosts to a total of 60-65 Gy are given to the primary tumor. The boost volume may be treated with a multi-field technique, perineal field, or an interstitial implant.

In cases where the inguinal nodes have been shown to contain metastatic disease, additional treatment using an anterior electron beam port is given to a total dose of 60-65 Gy.

Chapter 7

Genitourinary Cancers

THE BLADDER

The majority of bladder cancers are diagnosed in the 50-60 year old population. Frequently, these tumors arise as superficial lesions without evidence of invasion into the muscular wall of the bladder. The most common presenting symptom is hematuria. Dysuria and frequent urination are also common complaints. Risk factors in the development of bladder cancer have been identified and include cigarette smoking, exposure to aniline dyes, and chronic bladder irritation.

Anatomy

The bladder is composed of a muscular wall with the two ureteral orifices located posterior and laterally. The urethral orifice is located at the base of the bladder. The triangular area between the three orifices is called the trigone of the bladder. This area is one of the most common sites for carcinoma.

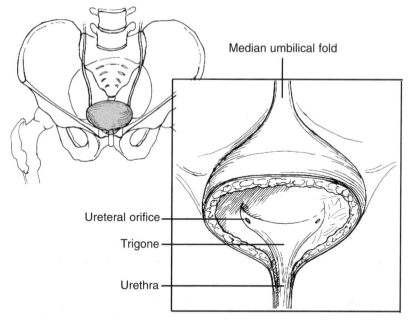

Median umbilical fold

Ureteral orifice

Trigone

Urethra

Fig. 7.1 Anatomy of the Bladder - Frontal Section

Routes of Spread

Carcinoma of the bladder can spread by direct extension into and through the bladder wall. If the cancer penetrates the mucosal surface of the bladder wall, spread through either the bloodstream or the lymphatics is possible. The primary route of lymphatic drainage is the external and internal iliac nodes.

Technical Aspects of Radiation Therapy

Primary radiation therapy plays an important role in the treatment of invasive carcinoma of the bladder. Definitive radiation therapy alone has been used in the treatment of bladder cancer with local control rates of 30-50%. More often radiation is combined with surgery or chemotherapy for improved local control. At present, the three treatment

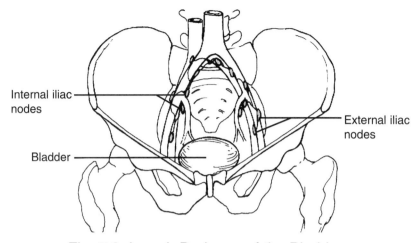

Internal iliac nodes

External iliac nodes

Bladder

Fig. 7.2 Lymph Drainage of the Bladder

alternatives include: 1) preoperative radiation therapy followed by cystectomy, 2) primary radiation therapy after a transurethral resection, and 3) transurethral resection, chemotherapy and radiation therapy. Treatment portals are similar for all three options.

For carcinoma of the bladder, a four field isocentric technique using high energy photons (6 Mv or greater), is recommended. At the time of simulation, the patient is catheterized and 15-20 cc of contrast media and 5-20 cc of air are introduced into the bladder. When the patient is supine, the air will rise, defining the anterior extent of the bladder. Barium is also inserted into the rectum. The patient is usually treated with the bladder empty to reduce the size of the treatment volume.

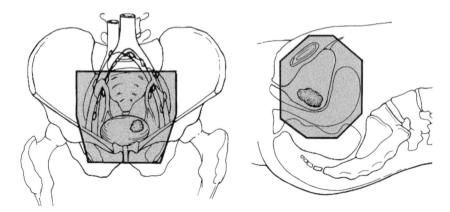

Fig. 7.3 AP-PA and Lateral Treatment Fields for Bladder

AP/PA field borders are as follows:

Superior - between S1 and S2

Inferior - bottom of the obturator foramen

Lateral - one to two centimeters beyond the bony pelvic side walls. (Field shaping is usually done around the femurs).

Borders for the lateral portals are as follows:

Anterior - usually extends 1-2 cm beyond the air bubble in the bladder. (approximately 1-2 cm anterior to the pubic symphysis).

Posterior - at least 2-3 cm behind the bladder and tumor volume. (A treatment planning CT scan can help better define the margin and spare vital organs and tissue such as the posterior rectal wall, small bowel and anus).

If the patient is a candidate for definitive radiation therapy, careful planning of the boost portal is done with the use of a CT scan, physical exam, cystoscopy and a urologist's diagram of the tumor. Careful planning can alleviate the need to treat the entire bladder and decrease both acute and long term side effects. Depending upon the location of the primary tumor, boost ports may be treated with lateral fields or AP-PA fields. Boost ports should be simulated with a minimum of a 2 cm margin around the tumor volume. Other techniques for boost treatments have been utilized and include rotational arcs, or an anterior port with lateral wedged fields.

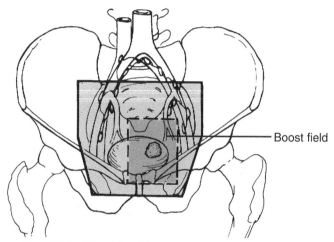

Boost field

Fig. 7.4 Bladder Treatment Boost

Dose

Preoperative radiation therapy is usually given via a four field technique to include the entire bladder and regional lymph nodes. Preoperatively, patients receive a dose of 45-50 Gy at 1.8 Gy per fraction via a four field technique. Surgery is then performed in three weeks.

For patients not able to undergo surgery or receive chemotherapy, definitive radiation therapy is an option. It is usually recommended that the patient have a transurethral resection of as much of the gross tumor as possible for best results. The bladder is treated with a four field technique to a dose of 45-50 Gy at 1.8 Gy/fraction. The tumor volume is then boosted to a total dose of 65-70 Gy.

Several clinical trials and protocols have used all three treatment modalities in the treatment of invasive bladder cancer in an attempt to preserve the bladder. Patients usually undergo transurethral resection of gross disease followed by two courses of multiagent chemotherapy. Radiation therapy is then initiated with single agent chemotherapy to a dose of 40 Gy. A repeat cystoscopy is preformed and if there is no evidence of tumor, patients are offered bladder preservation. They usually receive additional chemotherapy and radiation as a boost to 65 Gy.

PROSTATE CANCER

Prostate cancer is the most common neoplasm of men in the United States. It occurs most frequently in men over 60 years old. Carcinoma of the prostate accounts for 20% of all cancers and the incidence is increasing. The vast majority of prostate cancers are adenocarcinomas.

Patients may present with obstructive symptoms, an area of induration on rectal exam, or with an elevated prostate-specific antigen (PSA). PSA is an antigen found in seminal vesicle fluid and plasma which is produced by benign and malignant cells in the prostate. PSA is the best tumor marker for prostate cancer and is an important prognostic indicator. The level of PSA directly correlates with the patient's clinical stage, Gleason score, and treatment failure rate.

Anatomy

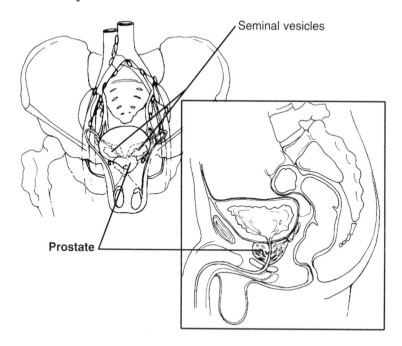

Seminal vesicles

Prostate

Fig.7.5 Anatomical Relations of the Prostate Gland

The prostate is attached anteriorly to the pubic symphysis. Superior to the prostate are the seminal vesicles and the bladder. The rectum is posterior to the prostate. Lateral to the prostate is the levater-ani muscle. The urogenital diaphragm is inferior to the prostate. The prostate gland is composed of five lobes. It consists of an anterior, a posterior, a medial and two lateral lobes. The urethra passes through the prostate gland.

The demarcation of the anatomical position of the prostate in relation to the bladder, rectum, and bony structures of the pelvis is critical in external beam treatment planning. The position of the prostate may vary in each patient.

Routes of Spread

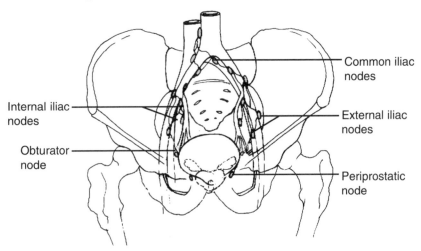

Internal iliac
nodes

Obturator
node

Common iliac
nodes

External iliac
nodes

Periprostatic
node

Fig. 7.6 Lymph Drainage of the Prostate

Prostate cancer may spread by local invasion, to involve the periprostatic tissue, seminal vesicles, bladder, and/or ureters. Prostate cancer can also spread through the lymphatic system. The first area of nodal spread is to the periprostatic and the obturator lymph nodes. Internal iliac, external iliac, common iliac, presciatic and presacral nodes may also be involved. Lymphatic spread increases with the stage and the grade of the tumor. Hematogenous metastases is seen with advanced disease. The most common metastatic site is bone.

Treatment

Treatment management options for prostate cancer include:
Observation - for early stage (A1-less than 5 chips on
                        TURP)
Radical prostatectomy - for disease confined to the gland.
(Not indicated in the management of extracapsular disease or positive nodes. Only 40% of clinically staged B2 tumors

are actually confined to the prostate at the time of surgery).
Implant therapy (I-125, Cf-252, or Ir-192 seeds)- for early
stage lesions (well to moderately differentiated
with less than 3 positive nodes)
External beam radiation - for all stages, including primary
therapy and palliation
Hormonal manipulation - for metastatic disease

Technical Aspects of Radiation Therapy

External beam radiation for definitive treatment of prostate
cancer is delivered in various ways. Improved treatment
planning techniques are presently allowing for smaller
fields, and may lead to fewer side effects and treatment
related complications.

The value of elective nodal irradiation is not certain. Initial
field sizes range from treating the pelvic nodes (from L5-
S1), to treating the prostate gland only in 3D conformal
therapy. Even though the initial pelvic fields may vary in
size, a four field technique is generally recommended. The
fields should include the prostate gland, seminal vesicles,
and the periprostatic tissue, with or without the regional
lymph nodes. A rotational field or multiple field technique
may be used for smaller treatment volumes.

It is imperative that the anatomical position of the prostate
gland, in relation to the bladder, rectum, and bony structures of the pelvis, be outlined by treatment planning CT.
When simulating the treatment fields, contrast materials can
be placed in the bladder and the rectum. A urethrogram can
be utilized to localize the inferior aspect of the prostate.
After localizing the prostate, and surrounding critical structures, a treatment field margin of at least 2.5 cm is placed
around all prostatic tissue. The posterior aspect of the rec-

tum and a portion of the bladder should be blocked without compromising the margin on the prostatic tissue. The bladder should be full during treatment to displace part of the bladder from the treatment field.

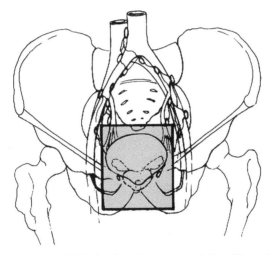

Fig. 7.7 AP Field for Cancer of the Prostate

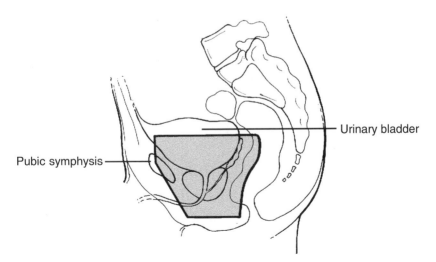

Fig. 7.8 Lateral Treatment Field for Cancer of the Prostate

Dose

High energy photons with beams of 10-18 mV are preferred. Generally, 45 Gy at 1.8 Gy per fraction is delivered using a four field technique. A boost is then delivered to a coned down field to 66 Gy at 1.8-2.0 Gy per fraction for tumors limited to the prostate (stages A and B), and 70 Gy for lesions that extend beyond the prostatic capsule (stage C). Postoperative doses are generally limited to 60 Gy to reduce morbidity.

TESTICULAR CANCER

Survival rates for testicular cancers have improved over the past twenty years, due to advances in chemotherapy. All stages considered, the overall survival rate for cancer of the testis is 80%. Although testicular cancer accounts for only 1% of all cancers in males, it is the most common malignancy in young men between the ages of 20 and 35. Testicular tumors usually present as a painless swelling in one gonad, and are often detected by self-palpation. Because 95% of all testicular neoplasms arise from the germ cells and the majority are seminomas, we have limited the following discussion to seminomas.

The periaortic and ipsilateral inguinal areas are usually treated with either a hockey stick shaped portal, or two abutting periaortic and iliac fields. The single hockey stick portal allows for ease of setup, and avoids any potential in overlap or underdosage that exists when treating two separate ports.

Anatomy

During the development of the fetus, the testicles form near the second lumbar vertebra. As their development continues, the testicles descend into the scrotal sac. The blood vessels and lymphatics follow the testicles from the lumbar region into the scrotal sac. There is an increased incidence of testicular neoplasms in patients with undescended testes. It is thought that these tumors are related to gonadal dysgenesis.

Routes of Spread

Pure seminomas, when detected early, are often localized to the scrotum. The primary route of spread is through the lymphatics. Due to the site of origin of the testis, the lymph nodes that are most commonly involved are the periaortic nodes along the lumbar vertebra and below the kidneys. On the left side, the primary nodes involved are the periaortic nodes below the renal vein. On the right side, the primary nodes are the lymphatics along the inferior vena cava. There can be cross-over drainage between these two groups of nodes. Therefore, both groups of nodes are at risk. In the pelvic area, some of the draining lymphatics terminate in the iliac nodes. Generally, only the lymphatics on the effected side are involved, unless there is a history of the patient having surgery in the groin or the pelvis which could alter the normal lymphatic flow. From the periaortic nodes there is usually an orderly spread to either the mediastinal nodes or the left supraclavicular nodes by way of the thoracic duct.

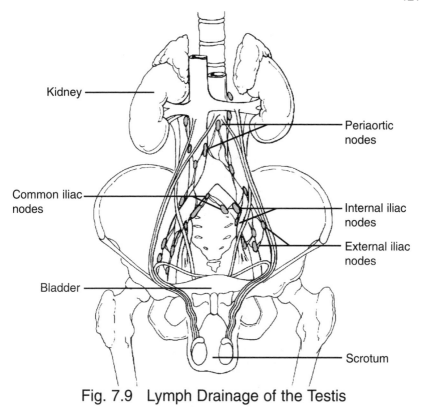

Fig. 7.9 Lymph Drainage of the Testis

Technical Aspects of Radiation Therapy

The treatment of choice for early stage seminoma, in which the tumor is limited to the testicle, remains inguinal orchiectomy with high ligation of the spermatic cord. Needle biopsy of the primary tumor, or orchiectomy by way of the scrotum, is avoided because of the risk of tumor seeding the scrotum and the subsequent need for treatment of the scrotum. Pure seminomas are extremely sensitive to radiation, and low doses of radiation can effectively eradicate these tumors.

The periaortic and ipsilateral inguinal areas are usually treated with either a hockey stick shaped portal, or two abutting periaortic and iliac fields. The single hockey stick portal allows for ease of setup, and avoids any potential in overlap or underdosage that exists when treating two separate ports.

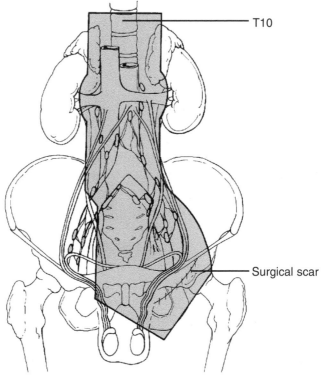

Fig. 7.10 Testicular Treatment Field

Borders of the Treatment Portal:

Superior - top of T10

Inferior-   bottom of the ischial tuberosity.

Lateral (periaortic region) - usually 9-10 cm wide, except at the renal hila where it may be slightly wider.

Lateral (pelvic region) - edge of the ilium to include the ipsilateral iliac nodes. The ipsilateral inguinal area and the surgical scar may be included, however relapse in this area is rare.

Medial border (pelvic region) - extends one centimeter over
    midline.

Custom blocks are used to shape this field and protect critical organs. This single field is treated as a parallel opposed
portal, and both fields are treated daily using 6-18 mV photons. If separate portals are used, the periaortics are generally treated with parallel opposed portals and the inguinal
field may be treated from an anterior field only, to a depth
of 3 cm anterior to midline. Testicular shielding should be
used. A lymphangiogram and IVP should be utilized to
ensure proper coverage of the lymph nodes including the
renal hilar areas. The lateral two-thirds of the kidneys are
omitted if at all possible.

Dose

Following surgery, the periaortic and ipsilateral inguinal-
iliac areas receive irradiation electively to a tumor dose of
25 Gy in 15-17 fractions. In patients with small metastases
to the pelvic or periaortic nodes, treatment portals are similar; however, a boost of 5 Gy to 10 Gy is given to the
involved nodes. For patients with bulky abdominal disease
or advanced disease, chemotherapy is given with good
results.

Chapter 8

Gynecological Cancers

CANCER OF THE UTERINE CERVIX

With the advent of the pap smear, the incidence of invasive carcinoma of the cervix has decreased significantly. Cancer of the cervix is now the sixth most common malignancy in women. Invasive carcinomas can be treated effectively with radiation. The treatment usually involves a combination of external beam and intracavitary radiation.

Anatomy

The uterus is located in the true pelvis, posterior to the bladder and anterior to the rectum. The three portions of the uterus are the fundus (superiorly), the corpus (body), and the cervix (inferiorly).

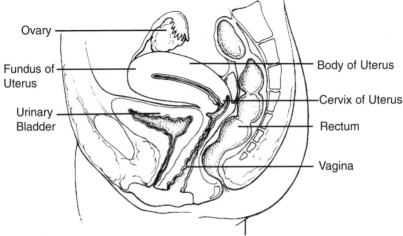

Fig. 8.1 Lateral View of Female Pelvis

Routes of Spread

Squamous cell cancer is the most common pathologic type of cancer of the cervix. The cancer usually begins at the endocervical canal, or at the external os (opening of the cervix). Initially, cervical cancer may grow downward into the lateral fornices (the superior most portion of the vagina). If the cancer extends superiorly, the lower uterine segment may be involved. The cancer may also extend anteriorly into the bladder, posteriorly into the rectum or laterally into the parametrium. The parametrium is composed of ligaments, connective tissues, blood vessels and lymph nodes that lie lateral to the cervix, and help support the uterus.

The cervix and uterus are fortified by a rich lymphatic system. The three most frequently involved group of nodes are the obturator, internal iliac and external iliac lymph nodes. The obturator nodes are a part of the external iliac chain and can be found against the pelvic wall, slightly above the acetabulum.

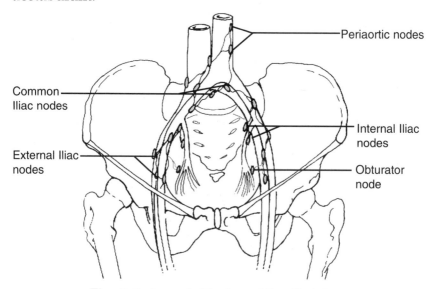

Fig. 8.2 Lymph Nodes of the Pelvis

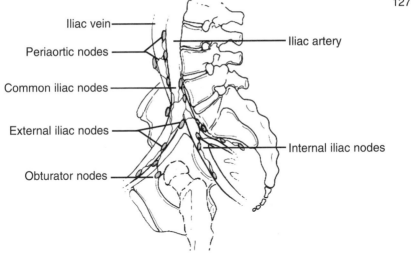

Fig. 8.3 Pelvic Lymph Nodes-Lateral View

The internal iliac, or hypogastric nodes begin at the bifurcation of the common iliac nodes and are located approximately 4-5 cm posterior to the obturator nodes. The common iliac and periaortic nodes are less frequently involved, but are at risk, especially with more advanced disease. The common iliac nodes extend from the top of L5 to the beginning of the internal iliac and external iliac chains, in the front of the sacrum.

Technical Aspects of Radiation Therapy

External beam is generally used in combination with intracavitary irradiation for cancer of the cervix. The role of external beam is to sterilize central disease and nodal disease that may lie outside the realm of intracavitary treatment. External beam is also used to help shrink bulky central disease to allow for optimal brachytherapy placement.

When designing the radiation ports, the known disease and potential sites of lymphatic spread must be encompassed.

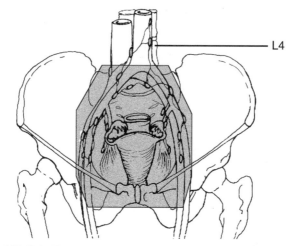

L4

Fig. 8.4   AP-PA Treatment Field for Cancer of the Cervix

The AP-PA Portal is set up with the following borders:

Superior - L4-L5 interspace

Inferior - the bottom of the obturator foramen (A radiopaque vaginal cylinder may be used to delineate
the cervix and to assure that the treatment port is
3-4 cm below the known disease)

Lateral - a minimum of 1 cm lateral to the pelvic brim to
encompass the external and internal iliac nodes.
The common iliac nodes lie medial to the SI joints;
therefore, cerrobend blocks may be used to
exclude tissue lateral to the SI joints.

If a lateral field is used the borders are as follows:

Anterior - encompassing the pubic symphysis

Posterior - split the sacrum. (Blocks may be added to
reduce the rectal dose and the dose to the small
bowel).

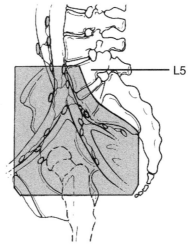

Fig. 8.5 Lateral Treatment Field for Cancer of the Cervix

Dose

Many different external beam and brachytherapy schedules have been used successfully. In most circumstances, the radiation oncologist will begin with external beam treatment. Most oncologists prefer beam energies of 10-18 mV. The higher energy decreases the dose to subcutaneous tissues and allows for either a four field or AP-PA technique. When using 4-6 mV beam energies, the four field technique is preferred to decrease the subcutaneous dose. The whole pelvis is usually treated with external beam to a dose of 40-50 Gy. An intracavitary insertion is performed either following external beam, or intermittently, to boost the dose to the central disease.

CANCER OF THE UTERUS

Carcinoma of the endometrium is the most common malignant lesion that arises from the female genital tract. The uterine cavity is made up of a mucous membrane lining (endometrium), a smooth muscle layer (myometrium), and an outer serous coat (peritoneum).

Routes of Spread

Most endometrial cancers are confined to the uterus initially. Spread of endometrial cancer is contiguous and involves the muscular wall. Once the smooth muscle has been penetrated, the incidence of lymph node involvement increases. The lymphatics that are commonly involved include the external iliac, the internal iliac, the common iliac, and the periaortic nodes. Transperitoneal spread may occur in endometrial cancer, as in ovarian cancer, and generally indicates more advanced disease.

Direct extension may occur and involve the cervix, vagina, bladder, and rectum.

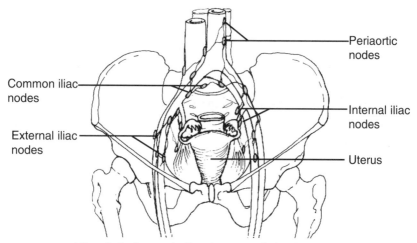

Fig. 8.6 Lymph Drainage of the Uterus

Technical Aspects of Radiation Therapy

Both preoperative and postoperative external beam irradiation and brachytherapy have been used in the treatment of endometrial cancer. Most oncologists in the United States prefer post-op radiation therapy, depending on the extent of tumor pathologically. Radiation therapy is recommended when the tumor extends beyond the inner one-half of the myometrium or when tumor extends beyond the uterus.

External beam treatment consists of whole pelvis ports. Beams energies of 10-18 mV are preferred, using a four field box technique.

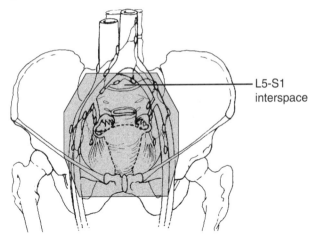

Fig. 8.7 AP-PA Treatment Field for Endometrial Cancer

Treatment field borders are as follows:

Superior - L5-S1 interspace, to include the common iliac nodes

Inferior - bottom of the obturator foramen or to include at least one-half of the vagina. (A radiopaque vaginal localizer is used to assure adequate coverage of the upper vagina).

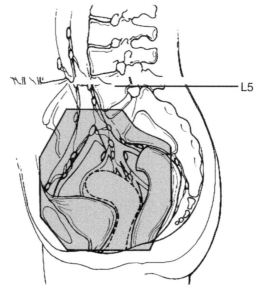

Fig. 8.8 Lateral Treatment Field for Cancer of the Uterus

Borders for the lateral ports are as follows:
Anterior - encompassing the pubic symphysis
Posterior - split the sacrum. (Blocks may be added to re-duce the rectal dose and the dose to the small bowel).

Dose

All four fields are treated daily with doses of 1.8 Gy to a total of 45-50 Gy. Brachytherapy may also be considered to the vaginal cuff.

CANCER OF THE OVARY

Ovarian carcinoma is not as common as cervical or endometrial cancer, but it causes more deaths than cervical and
endometrial cancers combined. Most patients present with
advanced disease. Less than one third of all ovarian cancer
cases are cured.

Anatomy

The ovary is supported in the pelvis and attached to the
uterus by ligaments. 80-90% of all ovarian malignancies are
epithelial carcinomas. The variety of histologies that remain
have a germ cell or stromal origin.

Routes of Spread

Epithelial tumors of the ovary often disseminate by shed-
ding cells that spread throughout the peritoneum. These
tumor cells attach to the peritoneal surfaces and form
micrometastases which continue to shed tumor cells. These
cells can flow from the peritoneal cavity through the
diaphragmatic lymphatics. Another common method of
spread is through the surrounding lymphatics. The main
lymphatic pathway travels along the ovarian vessels and
terminates in the periaortic nodes. A second route of lymphatic spread passes along the lateral pelvic wall and terminates in the external iliac and internal iliac nodes. Spread
through the bloodstream can occur, but is not as common as
peritoneal and lymphatic spread.

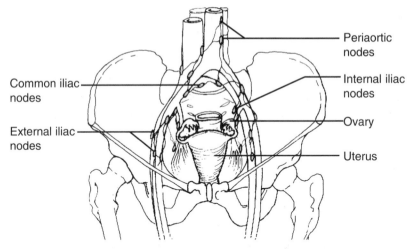

Fig. 8.9 Lymph Drainage of the Ovary

Technical Aspects of Radiation Therapy

The primary treatment for ovarian cancer is surgery. This usually requires extensive exploration and debulking of all tumor possible. Adjuvant treatment consists of chemotherapy. Radiation therapy is used less frequently to control microscopic or recurrent disease. Because of the pattern of spread in ovarian cancer, the entire peritoneal cavity (abdomen and pelvis) are at risk. Two radiation therapy treatment techniques have been used in ovarian cancer: open field and moving strip. Most centers have adopted the open field technique.

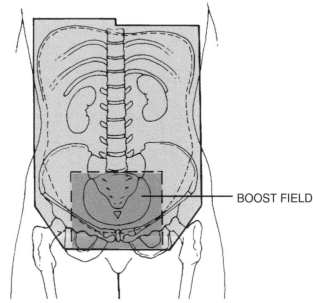

BOOST FIELD

Fig. 8.10 Open Field Portal for Ovarian Cancer

Borders of the open field portal:
Superior - 1-2 cm above the diaphragm
Inferior -   bottom of the obturator foramen
Lateral -   beyond the peritoneal line

Dose

The whole abdomen is treated to a dose of 25-30 Gy at 1.5 Gy per fraction. Liver and kidney blocks are used to keep the dose below tolerance. After the abdominopelvic irradiation, the pelvis is boosted to a total dose of 45-50 Gy. Consideration may be given to boosting a periaortic portal to 45 Gy, especially in cases with positive periaortic nodes.

Chapter 9

Pediatric Tumors

Major progress has been made in treatment techniques for pediatric oncology patients. Enrollment in protocols, combined with major advances in therapy, has resulted in a dramatic improvement in the survival and quality of life of these children.

Organs, bone and soft tissue are still developing in pediatric patients; therefore, late effects of aggressive therapy may be severe. Surgeons, medical oncologists, and radiation oncologists must make an effort to be conservative, without abandoning efforts to cure or control the tumor. For these reasons, pediatric patients should be enrolled on protocols in which the specific radiation doses and treatment portals are outlined. A multimodality approach is generally used to decrease side effects.

Typical treatment portals are presented in this chapter as a general guideline. It is important to consult current protocols for specific criteria.

ACUTE LEUKEMIA

Acute leukemia, a malignant disease of bone marrow, is the most common malignancy in children. It accounts for one-third of all pediatric cancers. Acute lymphocytic leukemia (ALL) accounts for 80% of all childhood leukemias, and is seen most frequently in children 2-10 years old.

Chemotherapy is the mainstay of treatment. Radiation therapy is used for central nervous system (CNS) prophylaxis, CNS relapse, or testicular relapse. Whole body irradiation may be used when performing a bone marrow transplant.

Anatomy

The central nervous system is surrounded by meninges which consist of the pia (innermost layer), the arachnoid and the dura mater. Cerebrospinal fluid flows inside of the subarachnoid space, which is the space between the arachnoid and the pia. The spinal cord ends at L2 in the adult, and the dura extends to S2. Depending on the age of the child, the spinal cord may extend below L2. Laterally, the sacral nerve roots extend radiographically below the L4-L5 vertebral bodies.

Routes of Spread

Acute lymphocytic leukemia is a disorder of stem cells and results from an overgrowth of immature lymphoid and myloid cells called "blasts" which replace bone marrow cells. Blast cells can infiltrate the periosteum, liver, lymph nodes, or spleen. The central nervous system is involved in 5% of children at diagnosis. The CNS and testicles are "sanctuary sites" at risk for harboring disease. When the CNS is involved the entire subarachnoid space (any area cerebral spinal fluid flows) is at risk.

Technical Aspects of Radiation Therapy

Cranial irradiation combined with intrathecal methotrexate is presently the standard treatment to prevent relapse in high risk patients. For CNS therapy the target volume for cranial irradiation includes the entire subarachnoid space and optic nerves.

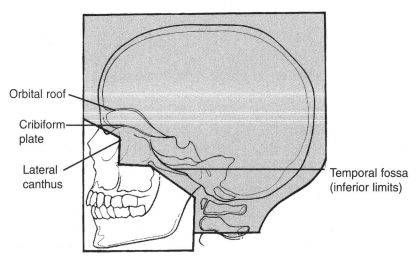

Fig. 9.1 Cranial Irradiation Field

The margins for the lateral cranial ports include:

Superior - fall off (Note: If matching to a posterior spinal port, you must allow enough fall off so that you can close in the collimator when moving the junction between the two ports and still adequately cover the top of the cranium without moving the central ray)

Inferior - to include the cribiform plate and temporal fossa subfrontally; to the level of C2 posteriorly

Posterior - fall off (a block can be added to spare tangential skin)

Anterior - fall off to cover the cranium

Proper attention to anatomical landmarks is imperative. Margins most likely to be inadequately covered include:

1) Cribiform plate - represents the inferior most site subfrontally and is sometimes difficult to include because of the proximity to the eyes.
2) Lower limit of the temporal fossa
3) Posterior retina and the optic nerve

To adequately encompass the posterior aspect of the retina and orbit while sparing the anterior half of the globe and lens, use a 4-5° gantry angle to correct for divergence.

Patients with overt CNS disease or CNS relapse require craniospinal portals. Most patients are treated in the prone position to facilitate daily set-up at the junction of the portals over the cervical spine. A board can be used to elevate the patient's chest and abdomen and their forehead is placed on a head rest to align the cervical and thoracic spine. Maximum chin extension should be achieved to diminish exit radiation through the mandible when treating the spinal field. The collimator for the lateral head fields should be angled to match the divergence of the spinal field. The treatment couch may also be angled to eliminate overlap from the divergence of the lateral head ports.

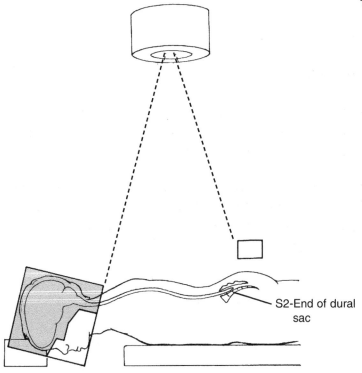

Fig. 9.2 Posterior Spinal Treatment Field

The margins for the spinal port are as follows:
Superior - junction of inferior border of the cranial port
Inferior - below S2
Lateral - the width should cover the entire vertebral bodies in the cervical, thoracic and lumbar areas. (A spade port to cover the SI joint area is used if there is sacral nerve root involvement).

The junction between the cranial and spinal ports should be shifted at least once during treatment to prevent under or over dosage at the junction site.

Testicular fields may be treated with photons or electrons with a single anterior field including both testicles and the scrotal skin.

(S2-End of dural sac)

Dose

Most patients are treated on protocol, but general doses are:
Patients who need CNS prophylaxis with radiation therapy receive 18 Gy at 1.8 Gy per fraction beginning on the first four days of consolidation therapy.

Patients with CNS leukemia receive craniospinal radiation with 24 Gy at 2 Gy per fraction to the head, and 12 Gy at 2 Gy per fraction to the spine. Standard chemotherapy is administered throughout the radiation treatments.

Patients who present with testiculomegaly at diagnosis generally receive 24 Gy at 3 Gy per fraction to the testes.

MEDULLOBLASTOMA

Central nervous system tumors account for 20% of the malignancies in children. Medulloblastomas comprise 20% of all brain tumors in this age group. The peak age for medulloblastoma is five years old. This tumor of neuroectodermal origin arises in the posterior fossa, principally in the midline of the cerebellum.

Anatomy

The posterior fossa has the following boundaries:

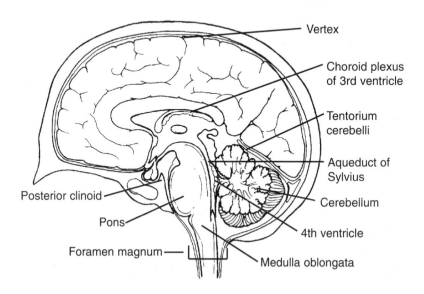

Fig. 9.3 Boundaries of the Posterior Fossa

Anterior - posterior clinoid
Superior - apex of the tentorium cerebelli (which is located
half way between the foramen magnum and the
vertex)
Posterior - posterior cranium
Inferior - occipital bone
Lateral - temporal, occipital, parietal bones

Routes of Spread

Medulloblastomas infiltrate locally and disseminate
throughout the neuroaxis. About 45% have spread beyond
the posterior fossa at presentation. These tumors can grow
into and fill the fourth ventricle or involve the brain stem.

They can extend supratentorially into the third ventricle or midbrain, or extend inferiorly to the upper cervical cord.

Another major route of spread for medulloblastomas is dissemination throughout the ventricular system and the cerebrospinal fluid (CSF) pathways. Microscopic tumor cells are often found in the CSF, while gross nodular seeding may be present in the third or lateral ventricles, cerebral subarachnoid space, or spinal subarachnoid space. Medulloblastomas also metastasize systemically in 6% of the patients.

Technical Aspects of Radiation Therapy

Surgery is used initially for tissue diagnosis, tumor debulking and decompression. The goal of surgery is maximum tumor removal. Surgery alone is not curative due to the tendency of medulloblastomas to seed through the CSF. Postoperative craniospinal irradiation is recommended in all patients. In young patients, whose age ranges from less than two to less than five years old, chemotherapy can be utilized to delay radiation therapy. In patients who have brain stem invasion, advanced primary tumors, disseminated disease, or recurrent disease, adjuvant chemotherapy is recommended.

When designing radiation portals, complete coverage of the subarachnoid space is imperative for irradiation of all CSF pathways. (For limits of the subarachnoid space, see the anatomy section for acute leukemia).

The patient should be treated in the prone position. The head is treated through two lateral ports and the spine through one posterior port. The borders for treating medulloblastoma are discussed in this section. (Details of a craniospinal set up are discussed in the acute leukemia - technical aspects of radiation therapy section).

The borders for the cranial port are as follows:

Superior - fall off (Note: you must allow enough fall off so that you can close in the collimator when moving the junction between the two ports and still adequately cover the top of the cranium without moving the central ray)

Inferior - to include the cribiform plate and temporal fossa subfrontally; to the level of C2 posteriorly

Posterior - fall off (A block can be added to spare tangential skin posteriorly. However, this would be contraindicated in a patient with a meningocele).

Anterior - fall off to cover the cranium

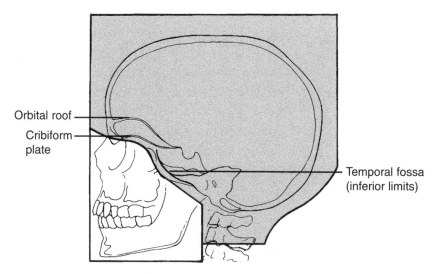

Fig. 9.4   Cranial Treatment Field

Unlike patients with acute leukemia, it is not necessary to include the retina and optic nerve.

146

Spinal port:

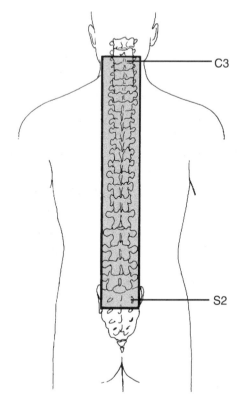

Fig. 9.5 Spinal Port for Medulloblastoma

Superior - junction of inferior border of the whole brain
port
Inferior - below S2
Lateral - entire vertebral bodies with 1.0 cm margin (a
spade portal is optional, but is not routinely done
because sacral nerve involvement is rare)

The entire width of the vertebral bodies is included to cover
the width of the spinal cord and the CSF pathways; and
also to permit symmetrical growth after radiation.

Cranial Boost Field:
The cranial boost field encompasses the entire cerebellum, pons and medulla, extending from the tentorium to the foramen magnum.

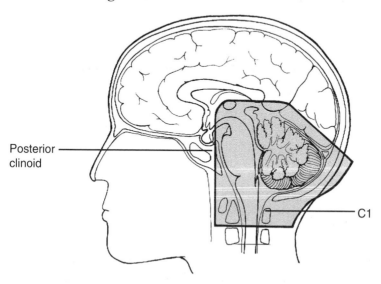

Fig. 9.6 Cranial Boost Port for Medulloblastoma

Superior - midway between foramen magnum and vertex, plus 1.0 cm
Inferior - bottom of C1
Anterior - posterior clinoid (attachment of the tentorium)
Posterior - behind calvarium

Dose

Generally, initial whole cranial doses of 35-40 Gy, at 1.5-1.8 Gy per fraction, and spinal doses of 30-35 Gy, at 1.5-1.8 Gy per fraction are recommended.

When craniospinal treatment is necessary, the gaps between

the cranial and spinal port should be moved two to three times throughout the treatment to prevent under or over-dosage at the junction site. The field borders should be changed by increasing or decreasing the field lengths without changing the central ray.

The posterior fossa should be boosted to 50-55 Gy at 1.8 Gy per fraction. Lower doses of 45-50 Gy have been used in children less than 2 or 3 years old.

Subarachnoid metastases should be boosted an additional 5-10 Gy.

EPENDYMOMA

Ependymomas occur in all age groups, but are most commonly found in children. In the adult, one-half of these tumors are infratentorial; whereas in children, two-thirds are infratentorial. Ependymomas represent about 5% of all intracranial tumors in children and are more commonly seen in males. We will limit our discussion to ependymomas of the posterior fossa.

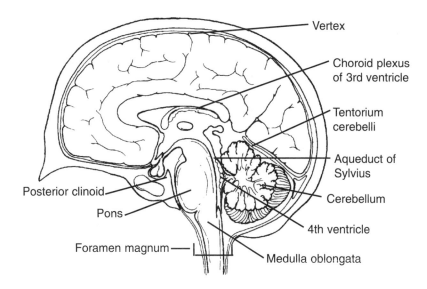

Fig. 9.7 Boundaries of the Posterior Fossa

Anatomy

Ependymomas arise from the ependymal lining of the ventricular system and spinal canal. Infratentorial ependymomas most commonly arise from the fourth ventricle.

Routes of Spread

Fourth ventricle ependymomas tend to spread locally, filling the fourth ventricle, or invading the cerebellum. They can also extend superiorly through the foramina of the fourth ventricle, or inferiorly through the foramen magnum to invade the upper cervical spine. One-third of the ependymomas arising from the fourth ventricle will extend beyond the foramen magnum. Careful attention must be given to the lower border of the posterior fossa portal, so that tumor is not excluded.

Ependymomas have been reported to seed the CSF (with an

overall incidence of 12%). CSF seeding is more commonly seen in high grade posterior fossa ependymomas. Presently, it has been shown that only 4% of patients with primary tumor control will seed through the CSF.

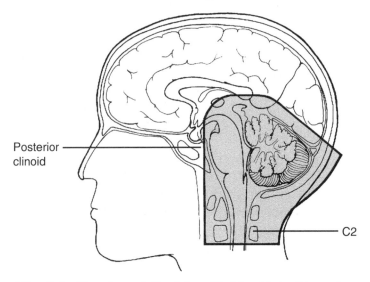

Fig. 9.8 Treatment Port for 4th Ventricle Ependymoma

Anterior - posterior clinoid
Superior - midway between foramen magnum and vertex plus one centimeter
Posterior - behind the calvarium
Inferior - C2-C3 interspace (with tumors that extend below the foramen magnum the lower border should be two vertebral levels below the preoperative tumor extent to a dose of 45 Gy)

Ependymomas are sensitive to chemotherapy, which has been used in some trials, but no definite benefit has been shown.

Technical Aspects of Radiation Therapy

Surgery is the first mode of treatment, with maximal tumor removal and preservation of neurologic function being the goal. Complete tumor removal is difficult because of the infiltrative nature of this tumor.

All patients are treated with postoperative radiation therapy. If the patient's myelogram or CSF cytology is positive at presentation, they should be treated with primary craniospinal irradiation (for portals, see medulloblastoma section). Some authors advocate craniospinal irradiation to high grade posterior fossa tumors with negative CSF. However, since local control has been the dominant pattern of failure in these patients, and because spinal dissemination is low in patients with good local control, the trend is to treat these patients with local fields only.

Dose

A dose response has been documented for less than versus greater than 45 Gy. The posterior fossa field is standardly treated to 50-55 Gy at 1.8 Gy per fraction in children who are older than 3 years old. The field is reduced off the cervical spine after 45 Gy provided that a 1-2 cm margin on the original tumor volume is maintained.

When treating craniospinal portals, the standard dose is 36 Gy at 1.6-1.8 Gy per fraction. The gaps between the cranial and spinal port should be moved two to three times throughout the treatment to prevent under or overdosage at the junction site. The posterior fossa should be boosted to a total dose of 54 Gy.

BRAIN STEM GLIOMA

Brain stem gliomas occur in all age groups, but are often found in children. These tumors comprise 10-15% of all pediatric brain tumors. Histopathologically, brain stem gliomas range from low grade astrocytomas to high grade glioblastoma multiforme. 38% present as high grade tumors, and an additional 10% are ependymomas and primitive neuroectodermal tumors. The most common presenting symptom is gait disturbance. Patients may also present with a headache, hemiparesis, strabismus, or cranial nerve dysfunction.

Anatomy

Brain stem gliomas include tumors of the midbrain, pons, and medulla oblongata. 50% of brain stem gliomas arise in the pons. The brain stem is a complex structure comprising multiple cranial nerves and long tracts. The most common cranial nerve abnormalities demonstrated are the involvement of cranial nerves VI and VII. The pons and medulla lie against the clivus with the junction of the cervical cord and medulla being located radiographically at C1.

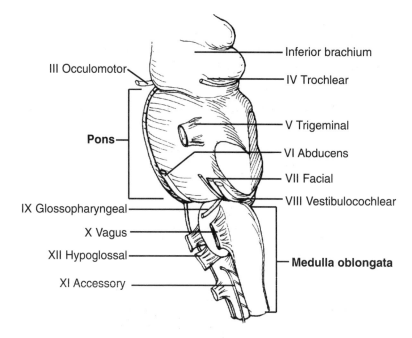

Fig. 9.9   The Brainstem

Routes of Spread

Brain stem gliomas infiltrate locally to involve the mid-brain, pons, medulla, brachium pontis or cerebellum. Subarachnoid spread has been documented in 15-20% of children. The more anaplastic lesions will have more extensive local invasion and are more likely to disseminate.

Technical Aspects of Radiation Therapy

Because of the location and infiltrative nature of these tumors, they are not usually surgically resected. However, surgery is indicated in exophytic tumors with extension into the fourth ventricle which have little brain stem infiltration, tumors of the cervicomedullary junction, or tumors with a cystic component. Biopsy is generally not recommended,

154

unless surgical resection is planned. Overall, the standard of treatment for brain stem gliomas is radiation therapy. Even though 15-20% spread through the CSF, a local field is the recommended treatment volume since most patients fail locally. Chemotherapy has also been used concomitantly in trials.

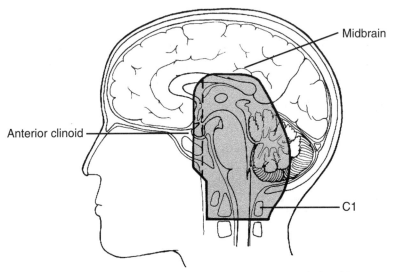

Fig. 9.10   Treatment Port for Tumor of the Pons

Treatment portal for a tumor of the pons:
Anterior - anterior clinoid
Note: Be careful to avoid the optic chiasm which usually lies anterior to the sella turcica. The anterior border may be placed at the "dotted" line as long as there is adequate margin around the tumor.
Superior - midbrain
Inferior - cervicomedullary junction (bottom of C1)
Posterior -mid-cerebellum

Important: The borders listed above are general borders that may need to be enlarged. An adequate margin must be placed on all areas of the tumor extension, as seen on MRI.

For midbrain tumors the entire extent of the tumor and a 1-2 cm margin are included in the treatment field.

Dose

Standard doses of 50-55 Gy at 1.8 Gy per fraction have been used, with a five year survival rate of 15-20%.

Presently, hyperfractionation trials are using doses of 70.2-78 Gy at 1 Gy, twice a day. There appears to be a slight survival advantage in the 70-72 Gy arm. An ongoing trial is testing a hyperfractionated arm of 70.2 Gy versus 54 Gy at 1.8 Gy, conventional fractionation.

RHABDOMYOSARCOMA

Rhabdomyosarcoma is the most common soft tissue sarcoma of childhood. The peak incidence is between two and five years of age, with a second peak in incidence in adolescents between the ages of 15 and 19. Rhabdomyosarcoma has been associated with various syndromes (neurofibromatosis, Li-Fraumeni syndrome), environmental factors, and anomalies. Two-thirds of rhabdomyosarcoma patients will be long term survivors.

Anatomy

Rhabdomyosarcomas are malignant neoplasms derived from embryonic mesenchymal cells. They may occur at any location in the body. Histologic subtypes include embroyonal, alveolar, pleomorphic and mixed variants. The embroyonal subtype accounts for approximately 60% of all cases. This subtype is most commonly found in the younger age group, and generally arises in the head and neck, or in geni-tourinary areas. The orbit is the most common site in the head and neck area. The alveolar subtype is more rare, accounting for approximately 20% of all cases. This subtype is more common in older children and generally presents in the extremities and perineal sites. It tends to metastasize through the lymphatics and overall has a poor prognosis. The pleomorphic and mixed variant subtypes are rare.

Routes of Spread

Rhabdomyosarcomas can spread by local extension, through the bloodstream, or the lymphatics. The lung, bone, bone marrow and lymph nodes are the most common sites of metastases. The incidence of lymph node metastases is dependent on the site of origin. The most common sites with positive lymph node metastases include the lower extremity (50%), and the paratesticular region (40%). Parameningeal tumors usually spread by intracranial exten-sion, and invasion of the base of the skull is common. Lymph node involvement with orbital tumors is rare.

Technical Aspects of Radiation Therapy

Multimodality therapy, including tumor excision and organ preservation, is presently recommended. The amount of residual disease is a prognostic factor. Total excision of the tumor is preferred to biopsy alone, depending on the site. After surgical staging, all patients receive multiagent chemotherapy.

Currently in the International Rhabdomyosarcoma Study (IRS)-IV, radiation therapy is recommended according to the patient's stage (which is based on the site of involvement, tumor size, and nodal status), and group (which is based on the completeness of tumor resection). The radiation therapy portals for rhabdomyosarcoma are site dependent. Overall, the recommended volume for treatment (in IRS-IV) includes the extent of the primary tumor and an adequate margin to cover the tumor and suspected areas of involvement. The tumor extent is determined at diagnosis for resected tumors (Group I-II), and after chemotherapy for incompletely resected gross residual disease (Group III).

If there is regional nodal involvement at diagnosis, the lymph node chain draining the regional area is included. Normal tissue tolerance shall be taken into account in all patients.

A parameningeal location includes involvement of the middle ear, nasal cavity, nasopharynx, paranasal sinuses or infratemporal fossa. Irradiation of this area requires careful planning. Because of its uniqueness, a treatment volume for a parameningeal nasopharynx presentation will be illustrated (Fig. 9.11).

A 2 cm margin is included around the primary tumor and the base of the skull. Regional lymph nodes do not need to be included unless they are positive.

If intracranial meningeal extension is present in continuity with the primary tumor, a 2 cm margin is placed on the intracranial disease also (whole brain treatment is not necessary).

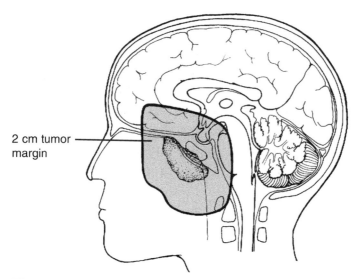

2 cm tumor margin

Fig. 9.11 Treatment Field for a Parameningeal Site

For a separate brain metastases the whole brain should be treated. If the CSF is positive, either craniospinal or whole brain irradiation and intrathecal methotrexate is utilized.

Dose

On the IRS-IV patients with an incomplete resection are randomized to receive hyperfractionated (59.4 Gy at 1.1 Gy BID) versus conventional (50.4 Gy at 1.8 Gy per fraction) radiation therapy, except for vulva and vaginal tumors which receive conventional fractionation.

All other patients receiving radiation therapy receive conventional radiation therapy to 41.4 Gy at 1.8 Gy per fraction. Radiation is to begin on week nine of chemotherapy unless the patient has a parameningeal site with positive CSF, bone or cranial nerve involvement, or intracranial extension. With the above findings these patients are irradiated on day zero with chemotherapy per protocol.

EWING'S SARCOMA

Ewing's sarcoma is the second most common bone tumor of childhood. It occurs more often in males (1.5:1) and is extremely rare in black children. A peak incidence is seen in the 10-15 year old age group. The most common site of involvement is the lower half of the body. It is frequently seen in the pelvic bones, femur, tibia, fibula, scapula, clavicles, ribs and vertebrae. The most frequent presentation is pain and swelling.

Anatomy

Ewing's tumor can be found in soft tissue, as well as bone. Although the disease can occur in any part of the bone, the diaphysis is more commonly involved than the metaphysis. The classical appearance on an x-ray is a diaphyseal tumor with involvement of the medullary cavity (onion-skin appearance), and an associated soft tissue mass.

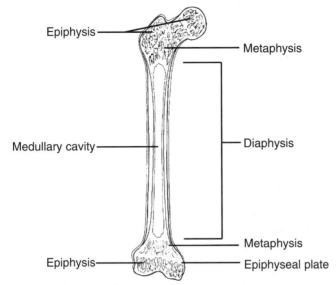

Fig. 9.12 Section Through Long Bone

Routes of Spread

Sarcomas most frequently metastasize through the blood-stream. 25% of patients with Ewing's sarcoma will have metastatic disease at diagnosis. The most common metastatic sites are bone or bone marrow, and the lungs. Less than 10% of patients have positive lymph nodes.

Technical Aspects of Radiation Therapy

Treatment generally includes a multimodality approach of chemotherapy, surgery and radiation. Surgical removal of the effected bone can be considered when:
1) the bone is expendable (fibula, rib, clavicle)
2) there has been a pathologic fracture, or an impending fracture (unless the fracture heals through induction chemotherapy)
3) in hand lesions, if wide local excision is not possible
4) when the lesion lies in the distal metaphysis in a child less than 6 years old
5) in large lesions that fail to respond to chemotherapy

In most cases, post-operative radiation therapy is recommended after conservative surgery. Patients with a radical resection generally do not need radiation therapy. In patients receiving radiation, strict attention to treatment borders is imperative in pediatric patients with growing bones; therefore, tailored portals are standard therapy.

When designing the radiation portal, the primary lesion and soft tissue component are included with a 4-5 cm margin. When the tumor is near the end of a long bone, the non-involved epiphysis can be spared to reduce late effects. For extremities, a lateral strip of normal tissue should be spared to prevent lymphedema. Also, the Achilles tendon should be excluded whenever possible because of late fibrosis that may occur after radiation.

For flat bones, i.e. vertebrae, the entire bone is included. For rib primaries with cytologically positive effusion, the entire pleural cavity is treated to 15-18 Gy at 1.5 Gy per fraction. Bolus should be used over the surgical scar, unless it is tangential to the radiation beam.

CT treatment planning and shrinking fields should be used when possible.

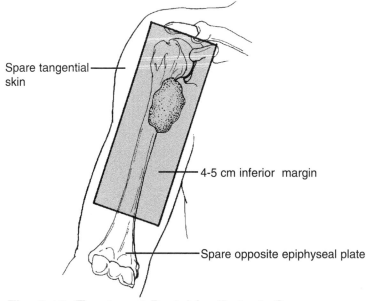

Spare tangential skin

4-5 cm inferior margin

Spare opposite epiphyseal plate

Fig. 9.13 Treatment Portal for Ewing's Sarcoma

Dose

These patients should be entered on protocol, when possible.

Doses of 30-40 Gy at 1.8 Gy per fraction have been used postoperatively for subclinical disease. Gross residual disease requires higher doses of 45 Gy at 1.8 Gy per fraction to the initial field (tumor and a 4-5 cm margin), followed by a 10-15 Gy boost to the tumor.

Many patients have a major reduction in the soft tissue component of their tumor after induction chemotherapy. Present trials with hyperfractionation have been basing the total dose on the patient's response to chemotherapy. The initial field with a 4 cm margin is treated to 36 Gy (1.2 Gy, twice a day). The final boost field, to include the tumor and a 2 cm margin, is treated to total doses of 50-60 Gy, depending on the patient's response to induction chemotherapy.

WILMS' TUMOR

Wilms' tumor, a malignant embryonal tumor of the kidney, is the most common malignant lesion of the genitourinary tract in children. It is bilateral in 5% of the cases. Wilms' tumor predominates in children less than five years of age and is associated with congenital conditions including aniridia, hemihypertrophy and genitourinary abnormalities. Wilms' tumors are divided into favorable and unfavorable histologies. The unfavorable histologies include anaplastic, sarcomatoid, clear cell or rhabdoid features.

Anatomy

Wilms' tumor originates in the kidney. The kidneys are located in the retroperitoneal space. The right kidney is generally 1-2 cm lower than the left because of the position of the liver. Radiographically, the kidneys are located between the 11th rib and the transverse process of L3. The renal axis

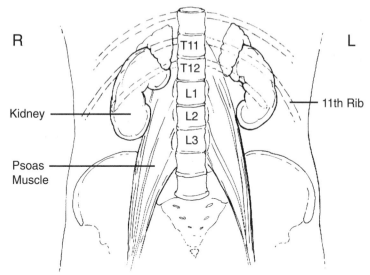

Fig. 9.14   Anatomical Relations of the Kidneys

is parallel to the lateral margin of the psoas muscle.

Routes of Spread

Wilms' tumor may spread through local invasion, lymphatic, or hematogenous routes. The most common sites for distant metastases are the lungs and the liver. Spread through the peritoneal cavity can occur if there is rupture at surgery. Rhabdoid tumors are associated with brain metastases and clear cell sarcoma may metastasize to bone or brain.

Technical Aspects of Radiation Therapy

Surgery is the initial definitive treatment in most cases of Wilms' tumor. All patients then receive systemic chemotherapy. Postoperative radiation to the involved flank is currently recommended in the following cases:

1) All cases of unfavorable histology (Stage I completely resected) excluding anaplastic tumors.

2) Unfavorable histology Stage II (microscopic residual dis-

ease)
3) Favorable and unfavorable histology, Stage III (macroscopic residual disease confined to the flank or positive lymph nodes)

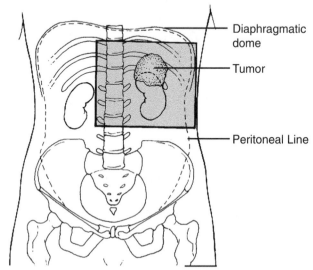

Fig. 9.15 Preoperative Treatment Field for Wilms' Tumor

Lateral -   outside peritoneal line
Superior - kidney and entire preoperative tumor extent and 1 cm margin (the field should extend to the dome of the diaphragm only in those patients whose tumor extends to that height)
Medial -   lateral to include entire vertebral body to minimize kyphoscoliosis and to include the paraortics (do not overlap contralateral kidney)
Inferior - kidney and entire preoperative tumor extent and 1 cm margin

If peritoneal seeding, diffuse spillage at surgery or preoperative intraperitoneal rupture is present whole abdomen radiation may be used.

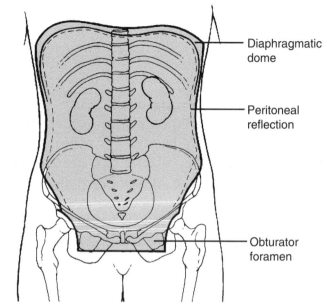

Fig. 9.16   Whole Abdomen Treatment Field

Superior - diaphragmatic domes
Lateral -   outside peritoneal lines
Inferior - bottom of obturator foramina (excluding
          femoral heads and acetabulum)

Dose

A greater than ten day delay of initiation of radiation after surgery has an increased chance of abdominal relapse.

For favorable histologies, 10.8 Gy is given at 1.8 Gy/fraction. Boosts are given to "bulk" disease (tumor 3 cm in diameter) including gross disease and 1 cm margin for an additional 10.8 Gy at 1.8 Gy/fraction. 4-6 mV photons are recommended. The dose to the opposite kidney should be less than 14.4 Gy and no more than one half of the liver should receive 19.8 Gy.

For anaplastic tumors a dose graduate scale is used, depending on the patient age, doses range from 12.6-37.8 Gy.

For whole abdominal treatment 10-12 Gy may be given for favorable histologies, with higher doses for unfavorable histologies. A boost dose to macroscopic residual sites is recommended to a total dose of 20-27 Gy, keeping in mind liver and kidney tolerance. In Stage IV patients with lung involvement, the entire pleural cavity is treated 10.5-15 Gy at 1.5 Gy/fraction with a boost to 20-24 Gy. The abdomen is treated according to operative abdominal stage.

Chapter 10

Soft Tissue Sarcomas

Soft tissue sarcomas are rare, and comprise less than one percent of all cancers. The most common presention is a painless lump or mass. These tumors can grow to a large size, especially in the buttock or thigh, before being diagnosed.

Anatomy

Soft tissue sarcomas arise from the extraskeletal connective tissues of the body (which include the muscles, tendons, fat, fibrous, and synovial tissues). Although they can originate anywhere in the body, approximately 60% will arise in the extremities. For this reason, we will limit our discussion primarily to extremity lesions.

Routes of Spread

Soft tissue sarcomas extend locally and spread along paths of least resistance. Fascial boundaries generally confine the tumor, forming a "pseudo" capsule. Hematogenous spread is common, especially with high grade lesions. The lungs are the most common site of metastasis, and are involved in 50% of the cases. Lymphatics are rarely involved in extremity sarcomas, except in the case of rhabdomyosarcomas, synovial cell sarcomas, or epitheloid sarcomas. The grade of the tumor is the most important prognostic factor in soft tissue sarcomas, and is a predictor of both overall and disease-free survival.

Technical Aspects of Radiation Therapy

Radical surgery, including amputation, has been the treatment of choice for soft tissue sarcomas. In recent years, radiation therapy has proven to be an effective surgical adjunct. When radiation therapy is utilized, less radical surgery is performed, and limbs can often be spared with successful disease control. Both preoperative and postoperative radiation have been used effectively. Advantages of each are listed below:

Post-op Advantages:
-Entire surgical specimen is available for histopathologic review
-Extent of microscopic tumor can be defined
-The surgeon does not have to operate in a previously irradiated tumor bed

Pre-op Advantages
-Allows for shrinkage of the tumor and a less radical operation
-May damage tumor cells on the periphery and prevent dissemination or spread of tumor in the operative site
-Treatment portals are usually smaller
-Pre-op doses are usually less

Treatment planning and careful limb positioning is imperative in the treatment of soft tissue sarcomas. The oncologist must define the muscle and compartment involved, as well as the extent of the lesion based on physical exam, CT, and MRI scans. The exact field margins, proximal and distal to the tumor bed, are controversial. Most oncologists plan a minimum of 5 cm proximal and distal to the tumor bed for low grade lesions, and up to 10 cm for high grade lesions.

The entire transverse extent of the compartment is generally included. Particular attention should be given to sparing a longitudinal strip of normal extremity tissue to decrease the complications of treating the entire cicumference of an extremity. Immobilization of the extremity is important and CT treatment planning is often used for planning of oblique and angled fields. Low energy photons of 6 mV or less are recommended for adequate dosing of superficial tissues. The entire superficial scar must be treated and bolus is used if the beam is not tangential to the scar. Regional nodal irradiation is rarely used except with rhabdomyosarcoma, synovial cell sarcomas, or epitheloid sarcomas.

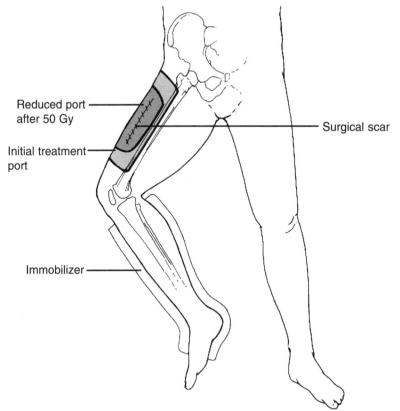

Fig. 10.1 Treatment Fields for Anterior Thigh Sarcoma

Doses

Pre-op doses of 50 Gy with 1.8 Gy fractions are generally used to the entire treatment volume. Total doses of 65 Gy with field reductions at 45-50 Gy and at 55-60 Gy are generally employed postoperatively.

Interstitial brachytherapy may be utilized as a boost following pre-op external beam and surgery.

Chapter 11

Emergencies

Emergent treatment is required for tumors that involve the spinal canal and result in spinal cord compression. Treatment should be initiated immediately to reduce the risk of permanent neurological damage.

Tumors that infiltrate the mediastinum and compress the superior vena cava can cause life-threatening complications. Immediate therapy is indicated to alleviate brain edema, reduced cardiac output or upper airway obstruction.

For both spinal cord compression and superior vena cava syndrome, it is generally recommended that treatment be started within several hours of the time of diagnosis, when the symptoms are minimal.

SPINAL CORD COMPRESSION

Compression of the spinal cord is most commonly caused by metastasis to the spine. Tumors most commonly extend posteriorly through the bony canal into the space around the spinal cord (epidural space). The four most common presenting symptoms of spinal cord compression include: pain, weakness, autonomic dysfunction (loss of bowel and bladder sphincter control), and sensory loss. Carcinoma of the lung, prostate, breast, and lymphomas are the most common primary tumors that may cause spinal cord compression.

Diagnosis of possible spinal cord compression can be made following careful neurologic exam, CT, MRI, or myelogram. It is imperative to document both the upper and lower extent of tumor involvement and cord compression.

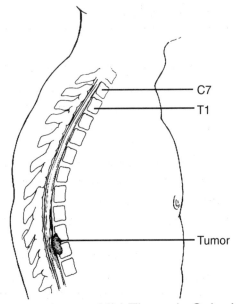

Fig. 11.1 Compression on Mid-Thoracic Spinal Cord

Treatment

The use of corticosteroids and radiation therapy play important roles in the treatment of spinal cord compression. Once the diagnosis of cord compression has been made, high doses of dexamethasone are recommended. Surgery is indicated when there has been no histologic diagnosis of cancer, or when x-rays demonstrate a collapsed vertebra. Under these circumstances, emergency laminectomy followed by postoperative radiation is recommended. Surgery is also indicated when there is evidence of recurrent cancer and the spinal cord has previously reached radiation tolerance.

Technical Aspects of Radiation Therapy

Following the administration of corticosteroids, external beam radiation is the treatment of choice for most patients. The patient is placed in the prone position, if possible, for simulation and treatment. After reviewing the imaging studies to determine the upper and lower extent of tumor involvement, a single posterior treatment port is simulated with a 3-4 cm margin above and below the lesion. Many oncologists prefer a margin of two vertebral bodies above and below the cord compression.

The tumor dose is usually calculated at a depth of 5-6 cm; however, this may vary according to the location of the cord compression. Lateral simulation films may be taken to determine the depth of treatment.

Treatment Borders for a Spinal Cord Compression:

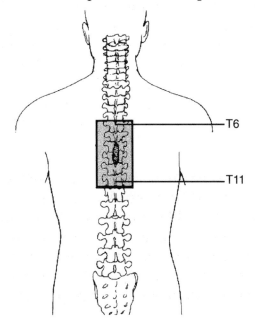

Fig. 11.2 Spinal Cord Compression Port

Superior - 3-4 cm above the cord compression
Inferior - 3-4 cm below the cord compression
Lateral - Typically 7-8 cm wide, but may vary according to
the lateral extent of the tumor.
Dose

The dose schedule may vary but typical total doses range
from 30-40 Gy in two to four weeks. The initial fractionation
schedule should be higher (3.5-4.0 Gy per fraction), for three
to four treatments in an attempt to maximize the response
as soon as possible.

SUPERIOR VENA CAVA SYNDROME

Obstruction of the superior vena cava by a mediastinal
mass produces a medical emergency requiring immediate
treatment. The superior vena cava represents the major
venous channel for return of blood to the heart from the
upper thorax, head, neck and upper extremities.
Anatomically, the superior vena cava is surrounded by the
anterior mediastinal structures and encircled by numerous
lymph nodes.

The two most common malignant causes of the syndrome
are lung cancer and lymphomas, accounting for 90-95% of
all cases. Benign conditions of the syndrome, such as thyroid goiter, account for only 2-3% of cases. The most common presenting symptoms of superior vena cava syndrome
are shortness of breath, facial swelling, distension of the
veins of the neck and thorax, chest pain, cough, and dysphagia.

Chest x-ray and/or CT scan of the chest will usually determine the location of the tumor; therefore, superior vena cav-
agrams are not necessary in most cases. Obstruction of the
superior vena cava may occur secondary to extensive compression by tumor or lymph nodes, or by direct invasion of
tumor into the vessel wall, with or without associated
thrombosis.

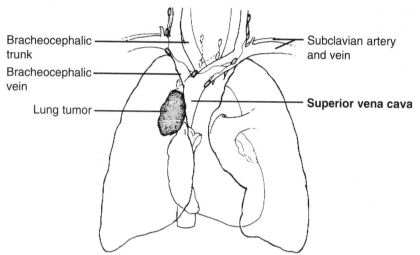

Fig. 11.3 Superior Vena Cava Compression by Lung Tumor

Treatment

Initiation of treatment should be immediate for patients
who are symptomatic, even though a tissue diagnosis has
not been established. Once the symptoms have been
relieved and the patient is clinically stable (possibly following only three to four radiation treatments), a thorough
work-up and diagnosis, including biopsy can be performed
safely.

External beam radiation therapy is initiated as soon as possible and is considered the treatment of choice.

Chemotherapy may be given initially for patients diagnosed with small cell carcinoma of the lung, who present with superior vena cava syndrome; however, this treatment remains controversial since small cell carcinoma is very sensitive and responds dramatically to radiation therapy. Many oncologists advocate the addition of steroids, especially in cases of acute respiratory compromise. Anticoagulants may also be used, especially if thrombosis is suspected and there has been limited response to radiation therapy.

Technical Aspects of Radiation Therapy

In cases with full blown superior vena cava syndrome and respiratory compromise, the patient may require treatment on a slant board or in a treatment chair. The treatment portal should include the primary tumor with a 2-3 cm margin, and the mediastinal, hilar and supraclavicular areas.

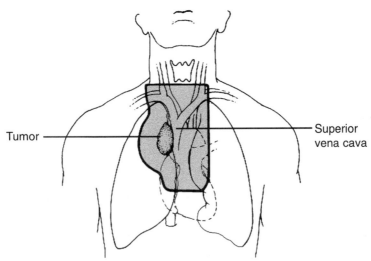

Fig. 11.4   Treatment Field for Superior Vena Cava Syndrome

Dose

Initially several high dose fractions (3-4 Gy) are given for two to three days followed by conventional fractionation of 1.8-2.0 Gy daily. Total doses depend on the exact histology of the primary tumor.

References

Ang KK, Kaanders JHAM, Peters LJ, Radiotherapy for Head and Neck Cancers: Indications and Techniques, Lea and Febiger, 1994.

Bentel GC. Radiation Therapy Planning, Macmillan Publishing Co, 1992.

Bentel GC, Nelson CE, Noell KT. Treatment Planning and Dose Calculation in Radiation Oncology, Fourth Edition, Pergamon Press, 1989.

Bedwinek JM, Breast Cancer: Post-operative Irradiation and Management of Locally Advanced Disease, ASTRO Refresher Course, October, 1993.

Breast Diseases, 2nd Edition, Eds. Harris JR, Hellman S, Henderson IC, Kinne DW, J.B. Lipincott Company, 1991.

Cancer: Principles and Practice of Oncology, 4th Edition, Vol 1, Eds. DeVita VT Jr, Hellman S, Rosenberg SA, J.B. Lipincott Company, 1993.

Cancer: Principles and Practice of Oncology, 4th Edition, Vol 2, Eds. DeVita VT Jr, Hellman S, Rosenberg SA, J.B. Lipincott Company, 1993.

Childrens Cancer Study Group (CCG-1901), Treatment of Newly Diagnosed Acute Lymphoblastic Leukemia in Children with Multiple Unfavorable Presenting Features, revised June 25, 1991.

Childrens Cancer Study Group (CCG-7881), Intergroup Ewing's Sarcoma, amended May 29, 1991.

Clemente CD, Anatomy: A Regional Atlas of the Human Body, 2nd Edition, Urban and Schwarzenberg, 1981.

Controversies in carcinoma of the prostate. Seminars in Radiation Oncology. Eds. Tepper JE, Hanks, GE, W.B. Saunders Co, July, 1993.

Cox JD, Moss' Radiation Oncology: Rationale, Technique, Results, Seventh Edition, Mosby Year Book Inc, 1994.

Fletcher GH, Textbook of Radiotherapy, 3rd Edition, Lea and Febiger, 1980.

Forman JD, Everything That You Need to Know About Prostate Cancer...But Were Afraid To Ask, ASTRO Refresher Course, October, 1993.

Fowble BL, Cancer of the Breast: Primary Irradiation, ASTRO Refresher Course, October, 1993.

Halperin EC, Kun LE, Constine LS, Tarbell NJ, Pediatric Radiation Oncology, Raven Press, Ltd, 1989.

Holleb AI, Fink DJ, Murphy GP. American Cancer Society Textbook of Clinical Oncology. American Cancer Society, 1991.

Intergroup Rhabdomyosarcoma Study-4 , July 15, 1992 revision.

Kun LE, Childhood Intracranial Ependymomas, presented at Tumors of the Central Nervous System, Harvard Medical School, Boston, MA, November 30-December 2, 1992.

Levitt SH, Faiz MK, Roger AP, Levitt and Tapley's Technological Basis of Radiation Therapy:Practical Clinical Applications,2nd Edition, Lea and Febiger, 1992.

Marcus RB Jr, Common Malignant Tumors in Childhood (Pediatric Sarcoma, Wilms', and Neuroblastoma), ASTRO Refresher Course, October, 1993.

National Wilms' Tumor Study-4, February 7, 1989 revision.

Netter FH, Atlas of Human Anatomy, CIBA-GEIGY Corporation, 1989.

Perez CA, Brady LW, Principles and Practice of Radiation Oncology, 2nd Edition, J.B. Lipincott Company,1992.

Practical Pediatric Oncology. Eds. D'Angio GJ, Sinnah D, Meadows AT, Evans AE, Pritchard J, John Wiley and Sons, Inc, 1992.

Radiation therapy for gliomas. Seminars in Radiation Oncology. Eds. Tepper JE, Larson, DA, W.B. Saunders Co, October, 1991.

Stryker JA. Clinical Oncology for Students of Radiation Therapy Technology, Warren H. Green Inc, 1992.

Wang CC, Radiation Therapy for Head and Neck Neoplasms: Indications, Techniques, and Results, 2nd Edition, Year Book Medical Publishers, 1990.

Illustrations as Slides:

Many of the illustrations printed here were originally used for lectures and handouts. They are currently compiled into a computer database. If you or your institution are interested in any of the illustrations in slide format for lectures or teaching purposes, or interested in customizing an illustration to your needs, please contact the following:

DWV Enterprises
3050 Hillsdale Drive
Augusta, Georgia 30909

or by calling (706) 721-2971

Please refer to figure and page number. Prices will vary according to image and order size.